"I've heard of M.E. before, but I didn't really know what it was, thankfully never had any friends or acquaintances who suffer from it. What an awful illness! This first-hand account was both fascinating and terrible, impossible for me to imagine."
Independent Australian review on Netgalley

"This autobiography particularly moved me. A poignant, captivating moving story. I hope she will release another book, her pen is addictive and her book deserves to be known around the world. There are never enough books like that."
Independent French review on Netgalley

"If you have chronic pain or an invisible illness, you will find yourself in these words."
Independent American review on Netgalley

"This memoir entertains and horrifies at the same time. The voice is spot-on. . . A fascinating and moving account of what it feels like for ordinary daily existence to become a struggle."
The London Magazine

"Jessica is an extremely talented storyteller and every word was a pleasure to read. Like many great writers Jessica draws you in with her imaginative narrative and keeps you engaged with every page—I found myself lost in her world."
The Mighty

A Girl
In One
Room

JESSICA TAYLOR-BEARMAN

Hashtag PRESS

Published in Great Britain by Hashtag Press 2021

Text © Jessica Taylor-Bearman 2021
Cover Design © Helen Braid 2021

A CIP catalogue for this book is available from the British Library.

ISBN 978-1-913835-01-9

Typeset in Garamond Classic 11.25/14 by Blaze Typesetting

Printed and bound in Great Britain by Clays Ltd, Elcograf S.p.A.

Hashtag PRESS

HASHTAG PRESS BOOKS
Hashtag Press Ltd
Kent, England, United Kingdom
Email: info@hashtagpress.co.uk
Website: www.hashtagpress.co.uk
Twitter: @hashtag_press

This book is dedicated to the millions suffering from Myalgic Encephalomyelitis across the world who are missing from society. It is for every person who hasn't felt heard or represented, those who have sadly lost their lives to the disease and for those who are being institutionalised simply for becoming ill.

Acknowledgements

This sequel has only been made possible through the incredible support I have received since A Girl Behind Dark Glasses was published in 2018. It was written over a long time due to my fluctuating chronic health and was edited throughout 2020 - the year a pandemic swept over the world. In the UK, a national lockdown was enforced to try and stop the virus spreading.

It was as if the whole world got a glimpse into the lives that chronically ill people live with every day. As an M.E. sufferer, lockdown is not a new situation for me. I've been living with it for years!

Without the incredible help from the NHS—even with the limited understanding of M.E. and often challenging admissions—I wouldn't be alive. I want to say thank you to Dr Paul Worthley who championed me and helped me more than I can ever express. My carers and nurses who have been with me in every emergency. Also I must thank my physiotherapist Clare and occupational therapist Diane who were so instrumental in my journey.

My husband Samuel has supported me, my health, and my dream of becoming an author, since we first met. Our beautiful daughter, Felicity, has brought so much purpose to our lives. Watching her grow up and being her mum is one of my greatest achievements.

Team Taylor and the rest of my extended family have been my rock. They've sacrificed so much for me. So Becky, Tom, Mum and Dad—thank you. I've been supported by some incredible friends, particularly Gail Gladdis who has been there come what may, Stewart Dimmick for always keeping me in check, and Sadie Hancock for being an incredibly loyal carer who then became one of my closest friends!

My incredible bedridden bridesmaid Alex Bliss.

Finally, I must thank the two incredible ladies who have believed in my vision from day one. Helen and Abiola thank you for your ongoing support and all the hard work you've put into this, whilst editing it alongside the fabulous Tiffany Schmidt.

Preface

I have been living in a recurrent nightmare of ill health since 2006. Its name is Myalgic Encephalomyelitis (M.E.). Just before my fifteenth birthday the M.E. Monster struck and changed my life forever. Before then, I had little understanding or knowledge of the chronic disease and how it affected the sufferer. I had only heard it being spoken about briefly in 2003 when I found out a girl I once knew had been diagnosed with it.

I was told in hushed voices by many people that we didn't 'do' M.E., and the 'joke' was that it stood for 'More Excuses.' I never saw the girl at my youth group again. It was like she had fallen off the face of the earth. Little did I know, a few years later, that would become my reality.

M.E. is a neurological disease that is invisible and still widely misunderstood in the medical world. In fact, it is so misunderstood that even doctors fight over—not only the cause of it—but the actual name of the disease. Many call it Chronic Fatigue Syndrome (CFS), but personally, I feel that that description is laughable in comparison to the daily suffering that I face.

Before the M.E. Monster inflicted chaos into my life, I had been the picture of health and happiness. My school report in 2005 read (in almost every subject) *'Jessica is an avid learner who is enthusiastic about everything she does - but she does tend to talk too much!'*

I had been the epitome of a 'normal teenager' living my best life. I had made no plans to leave it behind. Then, just like that, I lost it all at the tender age of fifteen.

The devastating symptoms destroyed my life. In a matter of months, my eyes became so sensitive to light that I couldn't bear to open them. I literally became a girl behind dark glasses. I lost all ability to function and was completely bedridden. I was admitted into hospital by the end of 2006; tubes were inserted to keep me alive and I faced a doctor who couldn't pronounce the name of the damn condition, let alone treat it.

I spent four continuous years in hospital on my own because I was deemed too unwell to be able to manage the stimulation of living with my family. Even though my health was fragile, the funding ran out for the hospital I was in. Then the argument mounted as to whether I would need to be moved to a nursing home at nineteen, or if my condition could be managed at home with community care. I desperately wanted to be able to go home and be reunited with my family. I wanted to live with my little sister Becky, who had been a child when I had left, and was now a teenager.

I learned a method to try to manage my symptoms, by pacing my energy throughout the day. I finally managed to make sufficient progress that it was agreed I could return home with twenty-four-hour care.

As my hope of being able to go home became a reality, I still held on to the dream that if I just kept fighting, I would be able to fully regain functional parts of my life that I'd lost. Then, just like that, the floor fell from beneath me and I was told that my bone density had silently wasted away, while I had been unable to move from my hospital bed, ruining my chances of being able to hold my weight. I was told I wouldn't be able to walk without breaking my spine.

The local health commissioning group decided they

could no longer fund medical treatment at the place I called Narnia and gave me the choice to return home or move into a residential care setting. In my mind it was a no-brainer; I wasn't going to spend my days in a care home. I wanted to go back to my real home and my family.

I eventually returned home a few months before my twentieth birthday. I tried to piece together what kind of life I was going to be able to live from the confines of my bed. I had replaced a bed and four walls in a hospital with a bed and four walls at home.

Despite everything, I chose to fight. I had to live. I was determined to make the best of it but I had no idea what challenges would come my way.

Welcome to my world of one room.

2010

CHAPTER ONE

The Journey So Far

Throughout my hospital journey with severe M.E. I was trapped in my hospital bed with excruciating pain; it was a lonely existence. No one understood. I needed a companion who knew the terrible ordeal that I was facing day in and day out.

But when I was first admitted into hospital, my exhaustion was so bad that I couldn't form sentences. It was like my brain was filled with fog and the slightest effort of trying to communicate was too much.

I used to be a very sociable person. I would often have half a dozen conversations going at the same time on my laptop, whilst still managing to talk on the phone. Even with the M.E. Monster controlling every aspect of my life, the person I was didn't change.

When I was at school, I was known to be fiercely independent and passionate about speaking up for those who couldn't stand up for themselves. I had no idea that I would have to become an advocate for myself and my condition. The medical world had very little understanding of M.E.; particularly with the severe sufferers. They often tried to suggest that it was a mental illness, despite the physical symptoms. Sufferers across the world were being taken away from their families and homes, when their only crime was that they had become seriously unwell.

Even now, over a decade later, patients are still suffering this neglect in the hands of health professionals who remain ignorant to this disease, which strips people of their lives.

CHAPTER TWO

Driving Home For Christmas

Acclimatising to life at home was more challenging than I had expected. There were new sounds and different carers to get used too. The M.E. Monster didn't manage change very well and I had been suffering with a flare up of all my symptoms since my journey home.

It was Christmas Day when the sensory overload completely overwhelmed me. This was the first time that our family had been able to celebrate together in *five* years. It was supposed to be a magical moment and whilst I was happy to be at home, it was hard to process my emotions.

I could hear all the festivities happening downstairs—the jovial cackle of Mum, my family singing along to Christmas carols, the smell of food—but I was alone in my room. I was too ill to be lifted downstairs and I was exhausted. All I could do was wait patiently to be spoon-fed a few mouthfuls of my Christmas dinner.

I had spent the past four years being miles apart from my family, but even though I was now in the same house as them, I still felt like I was far away. If Gran had been alive, I knew that she would have sat next to me and held my hand. She wasn't around the corner waiting to pop out and sing *Walking Through the Air* at the top of her voice. Her opal ring glistened on my finger; it was the last part of her that I could hold on to.

2011

CHAPTER THREE

Kneed To Get Better

The first few weeks of adjusting to living at home was both exhilarating and hard, in equal measures. Not having to wait for the weekend to have a visit from my family was just incredible! I enjoyed seeing my little sister, Becky, after school and hearing about her day, even though I was often too exhausted to be able to concentrate on what she said.

My older brother, Tom, lived ten minutes away and although he spent most of his time with his girlfriend, Jem when he wasn't working as a paramedic, I was able to see him so much more often.

Tom and Jem always seemed like the perfect match. It made me want to be in a relationship; to have someone who would care for me like Tom did for Jem. But it was highly unlikely that anyone in their right mind would take me on with all my health problems.

The challenge was trying to pace seeing my family throughout the day. I wanted to spend as much time as I could with them, but the M.E. Monster had other ideas. I was plagued with an exhaustion that meant I often didn't have the energy to hold a conversation. My muscles were weak and were unable to adequately protect my hundred-year-old bones when my carers tried to move me.

The first catastrophe hit me three weeks into living back at home. Becky rolled me on to my side as my carer took me off a bedpan. My quadriceps started to violently spasm. Suddenly, a searing agony in my knee—that I had never felt before—made me scream. I couldn't work out if it was nerve pain or if I had done something to my muscle. When I looked down to my horror I saw that my knee was completely out of place.

Dad ran into the room and gasped when he saw my dislocated knee. He rushed to his first response car and came back holding a cylinder and a mask.

"Alright darling, put this mask on. I'm going to give you some of this Entonox - it's known as laughing gas. It should take away some of the pain so I can put the knee back into place."

The gas immediately numbed the pain and once I had been breathing it in for a few minutes, Dad put his hands firmly on to my knee sending a shooting pain up my leg. There was a loud thud that made me shudder. I looked down and he had put my knee back in place! There were perks to having a paramedic as a Dad.

"Well done darling. I'm afraid we are going to have to get your leg X-rayed though."

My eyes widened at the thought.

"You have severe osteoporosis, so we need to make sure that your leg hasn't broken when the knee went back into place," Dad explained. "We will dose you up on pain relief, but you do need to get it checked."

The ambulance ride was marginally less challenging with

the strong concoction of medication I had been given. When I got to the hospital, I almost didn't notice Tom arrive in my cubicle. His bottle green ambulance uniform made him blend in with the rest of A&E.

The noise echoed around my head and even though it was dark outside, I needed to keep my dark glasses on due to the sensory overload. I fell into a restless sleep as the hubbub of the hospital became part of my dreams.

When the doctor came around and confirmed that my leg had not broken, I breathed a sigh of relief. Being back in a hospital had brought back terrible memories of being very sick. The M.E. Monster laughed at me as I remembered all the trauma of those years of hospital stays. It had a lot to answer for.

CHAPTER FOUR

They Know Best

I had been told by my care manager that a meeting—about me—was going to be held down the road at the doctor's surgery. They said I would be informed of the outcome, but they didn't need my parents to be there to advocate for me. The alarm bells already started to ring.

As far as I was aware, I would receive an email as to what they had discussed, so I wasn't expecting six medical professionals to knock at the door. Mum and Dad were at work so it was just me and Becky at home.

When they entered my bedroom, Becky instinctively squeezed my hand and gulped. It was overwhelming to have so many people staring down at us from the bottom of the bed.

"We're here to discuss how the meeting went," the care manager said. "I believe it went fairly well. We all know where we are at going forwards, wouldn't you say?"

Everyone nodded.

"We don't feel you're reaching your full potential. You've lost a lot of momentum in your progress since coming home."

Becky and I looked at each other, thinking the same thing. This wasn't what we'd expected to hear.

"I'm aware that there have been a lot of unforeseen circumstances and setbacks, but this isn't working out as well as we'd hoped. I know you feel there hasn't been enough physio to help you passively move but we all feel you should have progressed further. It's a difficult situation but we need you to go away for a couple of months again, to refocus, and then come back stronger," the care manager said.

What the hell? How can they have got it so wrong? M.E. is a chronic and fluctuating illness. It didn't matter how much I *wanted* to get out of bed, walk to the bathroom and have a nice hot shower, it was not possible!

The silence in the room was deafening.

"Where would I go? I mean, I want to stay here!" I said.

"But you must know that you are a detriment to your family by wanting to just stay here," the care manager said. "They don't have a life. Surely that's not what you want for them?"

I tried to hold the tears back, but the word 'detriment' stung me so badly.

"But we don't see it like that," Becky said to the surprise of everyone. "I want her to stay. We've only just got her back!"

"But that's the problem," the social worker said softly. "In stopping your sister from going and wanting her to stay, you're being a detriment to her, as she is to you."

"I want her here," Becky said. Her voice broke on the last word.

"Where would I go?" I asked. "I don't want to cause my family any harm."

I felt torn between being desperate to gain some independence to live a life that was more than just in this room and wanting to be with my family, where I felt safe.

"There are a couple of places we could look into. We could get you there for the beginning or mid-July. The only thing for sure is it definitely won't be Narnia—they are way above our budget," the social worker said.

There was so much I wanted to say but I couldn't get the words out. If I had to leave again I wished I was going to Narnia. At least they knew how to look after me. They eventually said goodbye and once the door shut, Becky and I looked at each other and began to cry.

CHAPTER FIVE

The Waiting Game

It had been three weeks since the multi-disciplinary team meeting and I was still waiting for the date for respite. They said it wouldn't be long.

Three weeks became six. They told me that I would go the following week. They said I needed to rest up so I had enough energy to survive the ambulance journey.

Eight weeks later, I was still waiting. Becky had started her first year of sixth form. She had been more anxious of late and I was worried about her. She said she was "just stressed" with her work, but I knew it was because she was worrying about me. I was even struggling to bend my legs on my own now. I just wished I could see the bloody physio terrorist!

Twelve weeks passed by and my pain was out of control. I was on constant adrenaline surges, and when the adrenaline went. . . let's just say it wasn't good.

CHAPTER SIX

Seeing Red

Respite was meant to happen in early July, but four months later I was still waiting for the authorities to give me the go ahead. Every week my health deteriorated due to the lack of input from my care team.

I hadn't seen a physio terrorist in months and my carer hadn't been signed off as 'safe' to do the passive exercises on her own. My occupational health therapist announced she was going to wait until I returned from respite to support me further. It was beyond frustrating for me but for my family it was soul-destroying to watch me suffer, knowing there was nothing they could do to change the situation.

My whole life seemed to be falling apart as the constant adrenaline of being told every few days that I would 'definitely be going next week' caused my body to crash. The M.E. Monster started to strip me of the few hobbies I had enjoyed with my limited energy.

My extreme fatigue meant I couldn't do any volunteering for my charity, Share a Star.

When I tried to distract myself by watching TV, I was plagued by the worst migraines. My family couldn't come into my room for long periods of time because the sensory overload made me physically sick. How was I meant to get through this without any help? Everything depended on this respite stay. My team had made that clear when they had told me I was a detriment to my family.

My phone pinged with an email notification from my care manager. My heart skipped a beat. This was it! I was going to get a date and finally get some help so I could get better!

Hi Jessica,
Well I've just received the news that we won't be getting you into respite until January. So I suppose you will get to enjoy Christmas with your family!

I read the email over and over, trying to digest the words, as the anger boiled inside of me. How could they? Why had I been left on tenterhooks for months whilst they continuously told me that I would be going next week?

I showed my carer the email, and she shrugged. "That's life."

"How can you say that? No one else has had to go through the hell of being told you are detriment to your family, your little sister being told that she is detriment to you, or that you have no choice but to leave your home. You haven't had your heart ripped apart and then been left to drown in the blood. You can never know that pain because it's not your life that is being messed with."

I started to cry. An anger possessed me like I had never experienced before, as I thought of the injustice for my family. I had spent years of my life being controlled by people, by the M.E. Monster, and I'd had enough.

"I need. . . to. . . get out of. . . of. . . this damn bed."

My broken body was too heavy to move, despite my best efforts. Becky ran over and put her body weight on to mine to calm me down.

"Let me go!" I screamed.

My carer walked away from me.

I then went for my hair, trying to pull it out to relinquish the frustration. So many broken promises, yet the multi-disciplinary team weren't doing a thing. They weren't suffering any consequences, but I knew that when my adrenaline went, I'd crash. My life seemed meaningless to them.

Becky tried to keep hold of my arms, as I thrashed about, desperately trying to get out of my own skin. Tom arrived home with Mum and ran up the stairs. My body was shaking uncontrollably and I just couldn't stop crying. Tom leant over the bars of the bed and put his body over mine to stop me from moving. I desperately tried to struggle but my body gave in and I let him hold me tightly.

"I can't do this anymore. I can't." My voice was barely comprehensible through my sobs.

"Yes, you can," he said calmly. "Maybe not today, but you will."

I cried for what felt like an eternity in Tom's arms, until I succumbed to the inevitable crash.

2012

CHAPTER SEVEN

A Horrible Hospital

I finally got the green light that it was time for me to go to the rehabilitation centre in Kent. As the ambulance arrived with Kip and Dad, Mum scanned the checklist of what I would need to bring with me. The suitcase packed with all my medications was larger than the one containing my clothes.

Once Kip had brought up all the equipment to safely transport me, everyone had to take a part of my body. Kip took my head, Mum and Becky took my torso, and Dad held my feet. They heaved my body around the landing and down the stairs to the back of the van.

As Dad grabbed one of the last bags that needed to be pack, Becky held on to my hand. "I just want you to know that I love you. I really don't want you to go," she said.

"I don't want to go either."

"I'm always here and even though I despise talking on the telephone, I'm at the end of the line."

"Right, we are ready!" Dad interrupted.

Becky and I gave each other one last look before she hopped out of the car and the engine roared to life.

We travelled for over forty minutes to get to the respite centre. I had been told that the hospital was one that specialised in neurological rehabilitation after a brain injury and that had immediately made me feel nervous. M.E. was not an injury to the brain so what on earth would their understanding of this mysterious condition be?

The ambulance trundled through the Kentish countryside, with Dad in the back and Kip driving. It didn't matter how many times I did it, being moved out of my room and into the ambulance was horrendous. My vulnerable body hadn't been in a different environment for so long that my eyes were scolded by the daylight.

As we came to the opening of the hospital, Dad nodded in satisfaction.

"It looks good, Jessica. I mean not nearly as good as Narnia, but it still looks nice. I was born not far from here. How have I never known of this place?"

"Describe it to me Dad."

"There are fields—lots of them. Oh, you would love this, there are even horses!"

I let out a gasp. When I had been well I loved going to the stables with my friend to look after the horses. I always found it remarkable how in tune horses were to how humans were feeling. They would nuzzle their heads into you if you were feeling sad.

The ambulance came to a halt as we arrived on the drive. Knowing that it was situated in such a place calmed my nerves and filled me with hope. Maybe this could be another Narnia?

Kip opened the back of the van and clambered in to help manoeuvre the trolley into the hospital. The receptionist directed us to a small room that had been prepared for my arrival.

It felt very clinical and the people weren't particularly friendly. It was probably a nice place; I had just been spoilt by Narnia in the past. There were very few places that could top that. Two people who looked like carers entered the little room to introduce themselves to me.

"Hi Jessica, we're the rehabilitation assistants on shift today."

"Oh, hi," I said nervously.

"What do you suffer with?" one of them asked.

"M.E."

I didn't miss the quizzical look they gave each other.

Once my parents had unpacked my belongings, their eyes lingered on my startled stare, as I looked into the emptiness of the room. Whenever I had gone to Narnia, they had always felt safe leaving me there, because they knew I would be well looked after. For some reason, this hospital had an eerie feeling like some of the frightening establishments I had previously been admitted into.

They held on to me before kissing me goodbye. They wouldn't be returning until the weekend, and as they shut the door behind them, I felt incredibly vulnerable.

The nurse came bustling in later that evening with a cocktail of medication to give to me. Within moments, she clumsily dropped the medicine and the 250ml of water down my front.

"For God's sake you moved!"

"No I didn't," I protested.

"You moved. I wouldn't have dropped them otherwise."

"I definitely didn't move because I can't move my body by myself."

She rolled her eyes. "Are you sure you really need to be on all of these drugs? I mean, it is a lot for someone so young."

"A doctor put me on them, so I think so," I said.

People querying the medication that had been painstakingly adjusted to my needs was always a sensitive subject, especially after years of disbelief regarding my extensive neurological symptoms.

Let it go, I thought, *it's not worth the trouble.*

I took a deep breath and smiled at her, praying that she would leave me alone.

The night was long; the M.E. Monster was let loose on my exhausted body. Each stimulation left me with a debilitating level of tiredness. Not only was I blighted with post exertional malaise from the journey, but my senses were also on overdrive because of the new surroundings. The unfamiliar smells, meeting so many new faces, and the bright lights were exhausting.

I was awoken early for breakfast by the rehabilitation assistants.

"Please could you help feed me?"

"Can't you feed yourself?"

"I'm sorry but I can't feed myself."

The other assistant begrudgingly started to push a spoonful of cereal into my mouth.

"Well, you need to give yourself a wash."

"I'm sorry, but I can't do that either."

"Why?"

"I haven't got the strength to do it." My cheeks flushed red and I looked down in embarrassment.

I got it; they called themselves 'rehabilitation assistants' because they were used to pushing stroke patients and other neurological acquired conditions to help them regain independence. These patients needed their encouragements. But this didn't help with chronic neurological illnesses that were invisible. No scan showed why my brain was malfunctioning and the agony that I faced in every part of my body.

"The doctor is coming to visit you, Jessica," one of them said to me.

When the doctor walked in, he immediately started to assess why I was there. You could see the cogs in his brain trying to understand why I was so disabled due to the M.E. Monster. How could somebody be that unwell due to M.E.? The one that they called 'Yuppie Flu' for decades? His lack of experience in M.E. was deafening.

"Jessica, I want to lower the dosage of the muscle relaxant that you take. I'm sure it's increasing your weakness and even your fatigue."

"But I'm on it because my muscles spasm so much."

"Let's see how it goes, I want you to try it. Now, on to your other medications. . ."

My eyes widened in panic, as he listed the medications that he wanted to change. It had taken years to get the medication right. As far as I was aware, I had come to this place for physical support from a physio terrorist and an occupational health therapist. The communications must have gone AWOL.

My decrease in medication started immediately, despite me voicing my concerns to the doctor. He wouldn't listen to me and the nurses all followed suit. The reduction in the muscle relaxant didn't cause me to become stronger, or less fatigued. Instead, my legs shook uncontrollably when I was moved on to a bedpan, and my pain levels rocketed. When the rehabilitation assistants tried to turn me and I yelped in pain, they ignored me and turned away, as if it hadn't happened.

I spent every night texting my family for hours on end. It had been less than a week and all I could think about was my desperation to get home to them. My family wouldn't hurt me like the people in this place.

ME: *Mum, Dad. They're taking away my medications. They won't listen to me. It is like they're torturing me. How can they do this?*

DAD: *Baby, what the hell? I will contact your care manager in the morning. I won't let this happen. They can't just take your medication away baby, they just can't. They can't do things against your will. Ring the buzzer and tell them that you're in pain and need pain relief.*

I tried to call a nurse but when she looked in, she quickly hurried away. The M.E. Monster cackled as it inflicted me with agony. I let out a sob; I had never felt so isolated.

CHAPTER EIGHT

"No Pain, No Gain"

The physio terrorist came to assess me the next day. He looked young and for a moment I felt hopeful that he hadn't been brainwashed with the 'let's keep pushing through the suffering' approach.

He moved my limbs, calculating the range of movement I had and worked out where my mobility needed to improve. He called the rehabilitation assistants in to view the exercises that he wanted me to do. My face dropped as he went over a vast array of exercises to help strengthen my muscles.

Did he not have any understanding of the condition he was dealing with?

Graded Exercise Therapy had nearly killed me on many occasions. It was the old school 'treatment' that doctors prescribed for M.E. sufferers. The idea was that you would increase an exercise by a percentage every week and you would have to do it, even if you were going through a relapse, or a bad day of energy and pain. M.E. had been plagued by misunderstanding, but how was it still the case in 2012?

After the physio terrorist had gone through the list of exercises, I began to crash. It felt as if I was being strangled by the M.E. Monster. My lungs felt tight, my limbs felt as heavy as if they were made of stone. This was all from *one* physiotherapy session. I had eight weeks to try and survive.

The complete exhaustion triggered a pain-filled insomnia. Even when I tried to speak up about how their 'treatment' was affecting me, no one listened. Despite my obvious suffering, the doctor wouldn't prescribe me any more pain relief. I was powerless to the ignorance of those who were in charge of my care.

"Bodies need stimulation Jessica." They would remind me every day.

It was hopeless. If I didn't keep going as they expected me to, it would look like I wasn't trying. It would become my problem if the treatment didn't work—not theirs—and I knew that this could affect whether I could get further funding in the future to go back to Narnia.

"Jessica, concentrate please," the physio terrorist would say whilst he manipulated my legs. "Come on, just another five minutes."

I thought about the plans for an extension to be built for me, but I knew this would only happen if I made progress here. So much was riding on this stay, and I didn't want to mess it up. I needed the council who had funded this respite; I was an investment to them. I wanted their help in the future. But with any investment, there had to be positive results. They wanted to see me being hoisted into a chair because that then gave them a reason to provide the equipment at my family home. If I was able to get into a wheelchair, that would give them evidence that I was the right person funding.

Thinking of my future needs was the only thing getting

me through the physio terrorist sessions, but by the end of the week, the exhaustion was such that I was barely conscious when he entered the room.

I had hoped that seeing how ill they were making me would give the team a reality check. However, my fears increased when I was informed that a psychologist wanted to see me the next day. The last time I had been seen by psychiatrist, who I had called Psycho Woman, she had been determined to get me admitted into a locked psychiatric ward in London. The only way we had managed to persuade her against it was through my diary that I had coded to my parents. It was only then that she believed that I wasn't suffering from severe depression. This time, I was on my own.

CHAPTER NINE

Psycho Man

When the psychologist entered the room, I knew that he'd need persuading to believe that I wasn't mentally unwell. It was Psycho Woman's sidekick, 'Psycho Man.' He sat by my bed, staring at me, waiting for me to talk. I held his gaze and smiled. I was in for a treat, I could tell.

"So, Jessica, I'm here to talk to you about your life, and what got you to this point."

"I became ill in 2006, with a virus, and I didn't really recover, which is when severe M.E. took over."

I had to think carefully about every word that I said. I battled with the tiredness that tried to prevent me from talking. I needed to make sure that he understood me.

"Okay, it's interesting that you use the words 'took over.' How did you know that it was going to cause something negative?"

Was he for real?

"Well, it wasn't a great thing to happen. I'm not negative about it."

"I see. Who do you live with at home?"

"My sister, Mum and Dad."

"What are three words that you would use to describe your relationship with them?"

He asked question after question, and my mind couldn't keep up. I tried to think of three words, but because it had taken me a long time to come up with some, it was taken as me avoiding the question.

"My relationship with my sister is happy, loving and funny."

"Why do you say funny? What makes you have a funny relationship?"

I tried to explain that she was an extremely funny girl. I told him a few of the gaffes that she would make and instantly regretted it. Psycho Woman and Psycho Man seemed to lack a sense of humour.

Before the session ended, he had labelled each member of my family with different ailments: Dad was angry and controlling, Mum was mentally unstable and overprotective, and Becky's behaviour was worrying.

He left me trying to understand what he had said.

How could he make such sweeping statements about people he had never met?

He returned a few days later, trying to see if he could find out the reason I had got unwell in the first place. He constantly assessed me on the language that I used, as if he desperate to find a flaw in my story.

"Jessica, I want to talk to you about the psychological part of an illness. You see, I honestly think that cancer is more of a psychological illness than many others. As soon as the word is mentioned, one thinks they must be dying and then it becomes scary. The word cancer fills everyone with an innate fear. How psychological is yours?"

For God's sake! Yet another person trying to insinuate that I was ill because of my psychological wellbeing. Don't they know anything? I took a deep breath and smiled at him.

"All diseases have a psychological element, but my M.E. is a neurological immune disease, just as it is described in the World Health Organisation. If it was just a psychological illness, then why am I not able to give blood or be an organ donor?"

He stared into my eyes, listening and nodding in various places. Once I stopped answering his question he left a long pause, wanting me to say more that would coerce me further into showing my psychological problems. It felt like a police interrogation; I felt like I would be locked up if found guilty!

CHAPTER TEN

What Value Am I?

A month into my stay, I received the news that my care manager was coming to visit me to view my progress. When she arrived, she looked less than impressed. The nurses and doctors acted differently, as they desperately tried to show her how much my health had changed in their care.

"So why has Jessica been having medication reviews? That is not something we agreed to pay for," my care manager said.

Finally someone was fighting my corner and telling the hospital that they had got it wrong.

"Jessica has been managing much more. The medication was just increasing her fatigue. She has managed to do physiotherapy sessions and we are looking to get her into a chair," the nurse explained. "She has even managed to feed herself a few mouthfuls. We have made huge progress with her functions."

The nurse looked at the rehab assistants for backup.

They seriously did talk a lot of a bullshit. I tried to speak to the care manager to tell them that the nurse was talking utter rubbish, but I was too exhausted to be able to communicate what I was feeling.

"So why does she look half dead if she has more energy? Why hasn't she received any hydrotherapy? That was the main reason we paid for this stay!" my care manager retorted. "Jessica's parents have been in touch with me and they're concerned about her wellbeing here."

"Oh no, there has never been an issue, we're just trying to get her body working. It's had years of deconditioning."

I wanted to interrupt but I didn't have the energy to concentrate on the conversation. I was scared of what they would say.

"If Jessica's health isn't boosted by this stay, we're going to have to look at a care home for her," my care manager said.

Suddenly everyone stopped dead in their tracks. Her words cut through me. She was meant to be on my side! She was meant to fight my corner. How could she? But I was alone and my body crashed from sheer exhaustion before I had a chance to challenge her.

Once everybody had left, I sobbed into my hands as the darkness engulfed me. I was no longer a person. I was a figure of money that had to be well spent. Figures don't need to be told what is happening to them, they just have to use the funds effectively.

As soon as I could muster the energy, I rang my dad. I was so scared about the fragility of my health and the situation I was in.

"I will get you home Jessica. I will send emails to every person that I have to. You just need to hang in there for me. I promise I will get you out," Dad reassured me.

"But what if they stop me from leaving?"

"I won't let them Jessica."

With the funding on the line, the physio terrorist came back with an even more intense exercise regime than before.

"It's all about progress and we need you to improve."

"What is progress though?" I asked him.

"It needs to be functional goals. We need to improve the strength of your arms so you can feed yourself and wash yourself. We need to improve your sitting in bed stamina because you need to be able to be moved into a chair when you go home—well—I mean, I'm not sure you could keep up the progress you've made here, even if you wanted to."

After the session, I laid motionless in the dark. How long could my body continue with this?

My phone rang.

"You may call me hero Dad if you would like!"

"What's happened?"

"You're coming home. I've had to make some agreements."

"Agreements?" I asked wearily.

"Well, you need to be in a bigger room that will fit your equipment in so you're going to move into our room, until we can sort out an extension."

"Really?"

"And we will continue your exercises when you're home."

"I'm definitely coming home?"

"Yes my darling."

A wave of relief came over me with such force that I began to weep uncontrollably into the darkness.

Dad arrived with Kip and the ambulance that was going to be taking me away from this hellhole. They swiftly moved me on to the stretcher and carried me to the back of the ambulance.

As soon as the doors shut and the engine started, I fell apart.

The hospital stay had been nothing short of traumatic. Psycho Man had mentally scarred me with his perverse ideology and the physio terrorist had taunted me, whilst the doctors had tortured my self-confidence by disbelieving my suffering. And for what? I was now in a far worse-off position.

The ambulance came to a halt and, as the doors opened, I took a deep breath. I was home at last.

CHAPTER ELEVEN

Olympic Glory

My health deteriorated rapidly following the horrible hospital stay. The fatigue and pain from the M.E. Monster felt like it was suffocating me.

In the mornings, I didn't even recognise who was in the room feeding me my breakfast. I came in and out of Limbo Land, the in-between world where I could hear voices but couldn't work out where they were coming from.

One morning, during my wash, I noticed a strange stabbing pain in my breast. It immediately made me put my hand to my chest to stop it. Then I felt it. There was a lump, that did not go away when I pushed on it. When I told Mum, she softly touched the area and her jaw dropped.

"I'm going to get the doctor to visit," she said urgently.

As the doctor felt my breast, her face said it all. She rang the breast clinic to arrange a screening.

Once we arrived at the local hospital, my heart started to race. My sister had accompanied me in the ambulance with Dad, and she gave my hand a comforting squeeze. My name was called, so we all entered the consultant's room.

"You must be Jessica's mum?" the doctor asked Becky.

Her eyes widened in shock, as she told him that she was my younger sister. He blushed and apologised profusely, before he briefly left the room.

"My God, I know I look tired, but I'm sixteen-years-old! How the hell do I look like your mum?" Becky grumbled.

"If you're the mum, who does he think I am?" Dad asked. "I don't know whether to be flattered or alarmed!"

"To be fair, I think he just thought that you were a random paramedic. I mean you are in the uniform," I said, letting out a stifled giggle.

Despite the ultrasound not showing up the lump, the consultant could still feel it, so he decided to do a biopsy. I felt reassured that it was being taken seriously, but I wasn't ready for the sting as the needle pierced into my breast.

"Sorry! We don't put local anaesthetic in for these types of biopsies. I'm sure that would hurt even more." He grimaced. "Okay, we're done. As soon as the results are ready, I'll write to you in the next few weeks."

The whole country was buzzing for the Olympic Games. It was incredible to see everyone unite. As I watched the grand opening ceremony, with Becky lying next to me in my bed, I felt like we'd all had our Olympic moments. My moment was when I finally learnt to speak again and move my body independently. It had taken me years of perseverance. But now I dreamt of having the strength to lift my head off the pillow. Maybe I could even leave my bed soon?

I watched the games avidly with Becky and we soon became experts on sports we'd previously not cared about. As I watched the cycling on the swelteringly hot last day, my body was struggling to regulate my temperature. One minute I was freezing cold and then within seconds, I felt like I was burning up. I suddenly felt overcome with an exhaustion that physically hurt, as I tried to process everything on the TV. The voice of the commentator swirled around my throbbing head. Then everything went blank as I was forced into Limbo Land.

"Jessica! Can you hear me?"

I could make out voices coming from somewhere far away. My body began to shake violently.

"Jessica! Oh my God! She's having a fit!"

A bowl of water was pushed off the bed by my uncontrollable limbs. I could hear my carer screaming Mum's name loudly.

Suddenly, I could hear Mum's voice, "She's too hot! We need to cool her down."

They undressed me, hoping I would cool down.

I was fighting the M.E. Monster to reboot my brain, but I couldn't find the right switches. It was like trying to find a needle in a haystack.

"Get a flannel that's not too hot or cold to sponge her down. If it's too cold, she'll go into shock," Mum instructed.

"I'm on it. You're going to be alright, Jessica," Becky whispered into my ear.

For a moment, I could hear the commotion of a crowd chanting. *Where was it coming from? Where was I?*

Finally, after a couple of minutes, my body stopped shaking and I became completely limp. Becky was holding my hand.

The M.E. Monster caused me to heave from the exertion. Searing pain hit me from top to toe, as all my muscles groaned pitifully. *What had just happened?* I slowly opened my eyes and tried to focus. Mum, Becky and my carer were in front of me.

Becky told me to squeeze her hand if I could hear her. I did and her face lit up.

"Well, that was a pretty extreme reaction to Sir Chris Hoy's last cycling race!" She laughed. "He won gold by the way. Britain's most-decorated Olympian!"

The next day my carer handed a letter that had the words 'PRIVATE AND CONFIDENTIAL' on the front with a NHS logo. I nervously peered at it, wondering whether this was the result I had been waiting for.

Dear Jessica,
We are happy to say that your results have been discussed at a meeting, and we can confirm that the lump in your right breast is not cancerous.

With a sigh of relief, I realised that we all have achievements. They might not ever be seen on an Olympic stage, but they are just as important. I managed to make the journey to the hospital and recover from it, so I was going to celebrate my gold win achievement as soon as the M.E. Monster allowed me to.

CHAPTER TWELVE

The World of One Room

I had lived within four walls for so long that it was my entire world. I couldn't even remember what it was like outside of it. To some, my severely restricted life was like a prison sentence, but I preferred to think of it as my very own world of one room.

The M.E. Monster could be described in many ways; he was the puppeteer who inflicted pain and suffering whenever he wanted. He was the prison warden and a torturer. He dictated every aspect of my life and took away everything that was important to me: my friends, my family and my education but even though he tried, he couldn't deprive me of my hope. He didn't have the power to take away my imagination.

My mind created endless possibilities; it set me free from my suffering. I could travel the world and live my wildest dreams. I could go from exploring the Great Barrier Reef to climbing Kilimanjaro in the space of a day. In my mind I was able to paint stars upon the ceiling, as if looking up at the sky on a crisp night. I could imagine that I was on a beach with the sun beating down on my face and the wind in my hair, but it was still a lonely existence.

Social media enabled me to escape. It became an instrumental part of my life because it gave me a voice. I found so many of my old school friends on Facebook and I connected with people all over the world on Twitter.

I joined a whole community of M.E. sufferers online who were all living in their own segregated lives. They became an army of support for me, as if we were all part of the same family. We understood each other's suffering in a way no one else could.

To my surprise, the connection to the real world through social media made me feel more alive than I had for years.

CHAPTER THIRTEEN

Please Don't Forget Me

2012 brought with it the horrendous news that a prominent member of the M.E. community had died at the mere age of thirty. Her name was Emily Collingridge and she had been the most incredible bedbound activist, fighting to raise awareness of this godforsaken disease.

Facebook was filled with tributes to her. Emily had spent all her limited energy on writing a book *A Guide to Living with Severe M.E.* The copy she gave me when I was in hospital became a lifeline for my family and carers.

But she died due to complications of the M.E. Monster that had blighted her life since she was a child. Emily was an activist until the very end and on her wishes, her parents released an appeal that she had written whilst on death's door. She had painstakingly typed each sentence on a smartphone over months. It was a haunting account that showed the chilling reality of severe M.E. and it demanded biomedical research and for an end to the ignorance towards the disease from the medical profession.

It was humbling to think that in Emily's darkest moments, she still tried to make a difference for other sufferers like me.

It was distressing to read all she had to endure in her short life I felt angry at the injustice of her death. It made me want to act in her name.

I wracked my brain trying to think of what I could do to raise more awareness. The problem that severe M.E. sufferers faced was that we weren't represented in society. People didn't know of our suffering because they couldn't see us. What could I do to change that? Then an idea struck me like a bolt of lightning: I could use my social media! I could use YouTube and create a film that gave an insight into my world of one room.

Over the next few months, I collected footage of every detail of my life: the triumphs and the crashes. It became a Team Taylor Production, as Dad would edit the video, then I would watch it back, and Becky would help me come up with punchy lines to go with it. I used my creativity to describe hidden parts of my suffering.

I wanted to show how I could at times become so unwell that I was forced into Limbo Land. People needed to see that I lived on so little energy that I required a carer to spoon-feed me my meals. I wanted to show how it was sometimes impossible to open my eyes because I was drowning in my own exhaustion.

The M.E. Monster had done more than just make me physically suffer and I wanted to show that. Dad found all the pictures of me before I became ill. There were photos of me with bright ginger hair from a hair-dye disaster, some of me quad biking through Scottish hills and others of me jumping on a trampoline. A lump appeared in my throat as I looked at them and remembered that carefree life that the M.E. Monster had taken from me.

The grief for the life I lost made me even more determined to raise awareness: my mind felt alive with ideas of how I could visually portray life with severe M.E. through my film. Whilst Dad edited the video on the laptop in my room, I found myself focusing on the slither of light that came through the crack in the curtain. It dawned on me how the world outside my window was so close, yet so far away.

It made me think of how much I missed being outside; lying on the grass in my garden and listening to the birds chattering to one another in the bushes.

"Dad?" I asked.

"Yes?"

"Can I ask you a favour? I want you to take a video of the garden so I can see what it looks like. I haven't seen it in six years and I miss it," I said quietly.

"Hang on, I've actually got one from a few days ago. All the buds are out." He fumbled on his phone. "Here."

As I watched the clip, I couldn't help but feel choked up. It was as if time had stood still. I could see myself in that garden, laughing as I played cricket with Tom and Becky. The relationship with my brother and sister was formed deeply through the times we spent together in that garden.

After a few more weekends, Dad and I managed to finish the editing. The film had taken so much of my energy but I felt proud and relieved that it was done. It was my story in a way that nobody had seen before.

In every process of making the film, I thought of Emily

and how much she fought to raise awareness. It was important that she was remembered and none of us were forgotten. We all had a voice that should be heard.

So, at the end of the video, I recorded myself and my friends from online saying, "Please, don't forget me," as a final nod to the bright light the M.E. community had lost.

Within minutes of sharing the video on YouTube and my social media platforms, it was being shared all over the world. The reaction to it was incredible! I received well-wishes from school friends, strangers and support from other M.E. sufferers.

A surge of adrenaline filled me as the views kept going up and up. Social media really could move mountains. Then came the crash. I was trapped inside a failing body, with intermittent paralysis. *Maybe the M.E. Monster was punishing me for making my awareness video?* Although I felt horrendous, the support that the video had generated gave me an extra ounce of hope.

In the film, I had shown what my greatest hopes were: to travel and have a family. I vowed that nothing was going to stop me. Those hopes had kept me going through my suffering for years, but the reaction to the video showed me that maybe the world was finally starting to take notice? It was beginning to wake up to M.E and see us.

CHAPTER FOURTEEN

The Close Shave

It was terrifying how rapidly my health could deteriorate. I started off with a slight pain in my stomach when I ate food and then it became sore to pass urine. Within hours the pain progressed to my kidneys and I became violently sick. The GPs had done all they could to treat me at home, but it became apparent that I needed urgent attention in a hospital, so an ambulance was called.

It was a Friday night and the hospital was pandemonium. The A&E department was packed with people who needed help, the corridors were filled with ambulance trolleys that had no place to go and there were ambulances that had been there for hours, queuing to get into the emergency room. Dad had come with me in the ambulance, whilst Becky and Mum had followed in the car.

We were moved to a small cubicle whilst we waited to see the doctor. Dad started talking to all the staff—many of whom he knew—whilst Becky and Mum fussed over me, desperately trying to get me to tolerate a few sips of water. But it was no use, the sickness continued.

The bright lights scalded my eyes. The noise from the other

patients and machines echoed painfully in my sound-sensitive ears. The M.E. Monster tortured me as the sensory overload penetrated my head so much that I couldn't focus on anything.

A doctor came rushing into the cubicle with a stethoscope around his neck.

"Hi Jessica, I'm one of the gastro doctors. We've found blood in your vomit, so we need to do more tests and take some blood too. Is that okay?"

I moved my head slightly to the side and nodded. It cost me all my energy to do that simple movement and concentrate on what he was saying. A nurse came bustling into the cubicle and tried to find a vein to take blood.

"Sharp scratch," and with that she pierced my skin.

She moved the needle around desperately trying to find a suitable vein. It hurt a lot, but I didn't even have the energy to make a sound of discomfort. After four attempts, she gave up and asked for a doctor to do it instead. A junior doctor hurriedly entered the cubicle. I knew as soon as I saw him he wasn't going to get the blood. He was far too complacent and my veins seemed to like to make the medics work for their money.

"Jessica, I'm confident that I will get it. I haven't missed yet. I promise that I won't need to do more than one attempt."

That one attempt failed miserably! There wasn't even a drop of blood when he took the needle back out.

I had always thought of my veins as rebellious teenagers that ran all the way through my body. They wouldn't cooperate unless they wanted to and certainly wouldn't be told what to do. I sighed as he tried again and again. The more he tried, the more beads of sweat appeared on his forehead. His cheeks became redder with each attempt, but after a few tense moments, he finally stopped and left the cubicle muttering that he had never had so much trouble before.

Another house officer came to try and get the blood. He tried to make conversation, as he pulled my arm tightly.

"So, why are you unable to get out of bed, Jessica?"

I winced with pain as my arm went completely numb. Becky explained about my condition.

"What is that?" he asked.

Becky gave a frustrated look and began to explain what M.E. was.

"Oh, is that the condition where you get a little tired? That fatigue syndrome thing. . ."

My face dropped as I realised that my health was in the hands of a doctor who hadn't even heard of the bloody disease that I suffered with!

"It's a neurological disease that is far more than just being 'tired.' It causes indescribable suffering and my daughter has been bravely fighting it for years," Mum interjected.

"So it isn't MS?"

"No, it's Myalgic Encephalomyelitis."

"But it's Chronic Fatigue Syndrome?"

"It can be known as that."

"We are taught that CFS is not a physical condition."

Mum let out an exasperated sigh. To be in the care of doctors who had no knowledge of the disease I suffered with was terrifying. I silently fumed at his ignorance as he turned his focus to my arm. No veins had popped up despite how hard he was holding it. He gave it a go and became frustrated that he'd missed.

"I'll have to get someone with more experience. I'm sorry that I hurt you." He left the cubicle to page another doctor.

A short while later, a female doctor bustled in and introduced herself to me. She had blonde hair in a neat ponytail and a South African accent. She couldn't have been much older than twenty-five, which felt strange, as it wasn't far from my age.

"I hear your veins are causing my colleagues trouble. I'll give it two attempts, otherwise we will have to look into other options." She sighed at the crash site that was my arms. "What the hell have they done to you?"

I looked down and saw that my arms were covered in red speckles that looked like chicken pox. She saw my look of alarm and reassured me that it was just my small blood vessels that had burst, where the tourniquet had been so tight.

"Don't worry, they'll repair. It just makes my job a hell of a lot harder. I'm not letting anyone else make such a pig's ear out of it." She oozed sassy girl power and I knew I was in safe hands. "I'm sorry if this takes a while. I will not be rushed because I can't fail. Getting your blood is the only way we can find out what's going on in your body."

She scoured my body for any hint of a vein, before she calmly announced that she was going to try in my foot. In comparison to all the other attempts that had been made, it didn't hurt at all. The blood poured out, which meant that it had thankfully gone into a vein. A smile appeared on her face, as she syringed out enough blood.

"We will get you better, Jessica. I guarantee that you're in the right place." She left my bed, holding the precious vials of blood.

Whilst I waited for the blood test to return, I was moved

to a medical ward. The only space was on a gynaecology unit, which was a part of the hospital I had not been to before.

"You really are trying to visit all the wards in this hospital." Becky grinned. "I mean if you were that desperate, I could've arranged for a tour of the place! In fact, I know what you can do, you know that book you were going to write with Gran? What about an essential guide to our local hospital? You'd be considered an expert."

I smiled but was too weak to utter a word. My struggling body had crashed with dehydration, despite the fluids that were pouring into me through a drip. I felt like a shadow of myself, with dark glasses shielding my eyes from view, even though it was late in the evening. I flinched with the noises of the machines, as Becky continued to comfort me by resting her head on my shoulder.

The nurse came around and introduced herself to me as Joy. "Jessica, I'll be looking after you tonight. Visiting times have ended though, so I'll have to ask your family to leave."

I tried to look brave and nodded encouragingly at Mum and Becky, who desperately wanted to stay by my side. Dad squeezed Becky's shoulder and guided her to the door.

I suddenly felt alone. The night was long, as I watched the time slowly pass. I drifted in and out of sleep before I started being sick. I pressed the buzzer for help, but the nurses were too busy to answer it. I laid in my own vomit for over an hour before they were able to clean me up. I just wanted to go home.

In the morning I was relieved when my carer from home arrived on the ward to be my one-to-one support. She sat by my side and kept trying to feed me sips of water and tiny bits of a cereal bar that she had bought from the shop. I was so hungry and thirsty, but I couldn't keep anything down.

I was taken for multiple tests, from X-rays to CT scans, and more blood tests to see if there was a blockage that was causing the sickness. But they all came back negative. *What was wrong with me?* I was a medical mystery that was confusing the doctors immensely.

I was moved to a gastro ward for more investigations. My M.E. symptoms were out of control because I couldn't keep any of my medications down. The Monster was torturing me with constant neuropathic pain throughout my body, pushing me to the edge.

The new ward was much busier and louder than the one I had previously been on. My senses were in overdrive as the hustle and bustle of thirty patients, nurses, and doctors filled my ears, but I still felt alone.

I let out a sigh of relief as Mum and Becky arrived at the opening of the cubicle. They had brought me a magazine to read through that had all the latest fashion styles, alongside the latest celebrity gossip.

"I mean really, does anybody actually care about the latest thing Jordan is wearing?" whispered Becky, as she skimmed through it.

One of the doctors came into the little cubicle to take more blood.

I sighed and wondered how many more tests I could possibly have. My arms looked like I was in *The Simpsons* but with a bad case of measles. They were completely yellow with bruising that made them painful to touch.

My family and carers updated my social media for me.

The internet had brought me close to so many chronically ill sufferers from around the world, who became my friends. One was called Blissy—her surname was Bliss—and she sent me audio messages and posted presents to me. She even kept an eye on how Becky and Mum were coping, whilst I was not with them.

My body was weakening more and more every day that I was on the gastro ward. My parents spent all their time arguing with the doctors to try and get them to do something. I was reminded very much of the horrific time I was first admitted into hospital in 2006. Six years later, and to my despair, history was repeating itself.

The consultant on the ward came to discuss my options. He was a short, older doctor, with a stern face.

"I think we need to look at artificially feeding you, Jessica, because your weight has plummeted. We can either use a naso-gastric tube or a PEG. We can look at giving you nutrition through your veins, depending on what's the best option for you."

I had been free from being fed via a tube for four years. It felt like a huge step backwards. I felt like a failure.

CHAPTER FIFTEEN

Feed Me!

On request from the consultant, a dietician visited me and made the decision that I needed to have a naso-gastric tube fitted immediately. The level of fatigue that I felt was so immense that I couldn't even make an expression: I just laid there looking vegetated. She was alarmed at how poorly I was and could see that I was dangerously malnourished.

The nutritional matron came to place the tube up my nose and into my stomach. I had forgotten how uncomfortable those bloody things were. The discomfort started as soon as the guiding wire had reached the top of my nostril. I kept trying to swallow, but instead my body contorted, as I began to heave. Once the tube was in place securely, I crashed into Limbo Land. The matron's voice and the noise of the ward echoed around my head, but I couldn't focus. Then I was out.

I was woken by the sound of a machine pumping a soya feed into my NG tube. My nostril was still painfully throbbing where the new tube was situated. I vowed to myself that it was only going to be a temporary measure and that I'd be enjoying a roast dinner with my family soon.

The doctors made a plan that the nurses would administer

different injections throughout the day to try and control the sickness, in the hope that I would then be able to start eating. They didn't understand that my M.E. had now relapsed, or that I didn't have the energy to swallow any food.

The nurses' lack of organisation made the matter worse. They often ran out of my feed and forgot to give me the anti-emetics in time for me to eat, leaving me with no nutrition. I was losing more weight and getting weaker as the days went on.

One evening a night nurse came into my cubicle. She didn't acknowledge me as she syringed different liquids into my tube. *Must be the medication*, I thought. I felt so exhausted that I had to close my eyes. I didn't know that it was possible to feel so fatigued that it was a struggle to find the energy to even take a breath. This was hopeless.

The nurse left and as I fell into a disturbed sleep, I began to dream. A woman was standing by the door that was opposite to my bed. I recognised her but couldn't work out why. She looked effervescent as she smiled at me. Then I realised that it was my gran! My beautiful gran. I just wanted to hold her hand and feel her arms around me.

I tried to get up out of the bed to see her, but even in my dreams, my body remained stiff. It had been over four years since I had last seen her and even then, I hadn't been able to hug her because my body was so painful. I watched as my dream brought her closer to me.

I could hear a voice in the distance urgently calling my name. *Who was it?* I groggily began to force my eyes open.

"Jessica!" My carer let out a sigh of relief as I came to. "I thought you were gone. I really did. You just wouldn't stir.

God, I was so sca—" She stopped mid-sentence and her face fell. "Your tube! My God! The feed is everywhere."

Somehow the floor was drenched in the feed that should have been going into my stomach. When my carer reached the machine with my feed hanging up, she realised it hadn't been connected to my tube.

She called my family immediately and they rushed in. The notes by the end of my bed stated that the tube had been checked every two hours, but there was no way this was true. They hadn't come in to make sure I was okay all night.

"How has this happened? They didn't even check on you! I can't leave you here. We've got to get you out of here because otherwise this place is going to kill you," Mum said. "I've nearly lost you too many times and I can't go through it again. I just can't."

Dad held her tight in his arms. It was breaking them. I didn't want them to suffer any more for me.

I've got this, I told myself. *I need to get home.*

In the evening Dad managed to persuade Mum to leave me after visiting time, before the staff forced her out. I tried to smile and be brave to reassure her that I was going to be okay. Less than an hour later, the night nurse came in.

"I'm afraid we don't have any of your night medications. The day nurses must have forgotten to order it."

My mouth dropped open as I contemplated having to spend a night without any pain or sleeping medication.

"Maybe you can ring your parents and see if they can bring some in? Otherwise you'll have to go without."

I cried down the phone to my parents, pleading with them to bring the medications.

"It's a hospital, for God's sake. How on earth do they not have medication?" asked Dad. "Don't worry, I'll bring in your medication, but this is farcical. What do I need to do to get people to care for you on this ward? I'll take this to the Care Quality Commission, mark my words."

CHAPTER SIXTEEN

Escape to the Chateau

Over the next few weeks, my parents fought for a plan to be put in place for me to be nursed at home. Dad came to every ward round before darting off to work, whilst Mum and Becky spent all day looking after me.

At the weekend Tom came to see me. He'd recently moved to Basingstoke to live with Jem, so alongside his crazy shift work, I didn't get to see him much. He asked to bring one of his closest friends with him. Stewie was also a paramedic and had a dark sense of humour. He appeared very shy and socially awkward when he walked in. He was shorter than Tom and stood behind him, emphasising the difference in height. At first, he struggled to give me a drink from my beaker.

"Jessica, this is Stewie. He's going to be there for you when I'm not able to be."

"I'm not used to looking at girls in their beds, let alone feeding them!" Stewie groaned.

"Mate, you're a paramedic. You see plenty of them!" Tom laughed.

"Yeah that's true. But they aren't my best friend's sister. I feel a newfound responsibility to not mess up."

With that, the water poured down my neck rather than my mouth, and he swore under his breath.

"Sorry! See what I mean?" He sighed. "I'll come and visit you at home Jessica, every week if I have to, as this man has abandoned us for Jem! You need a big brother and I'm happy to take over!" Stewie pointed at Tom. "Only kidding mate. You can't help falling head over heels in love with her. She's a good 'un."

"But you guys, I want someone! I'm alone and I would love to have someone who loves me," I moaned.

"Mate, we love you! You need to focus on getting well enough that you can leave this awful ward, okay?" Tom said.

"I will find you a guy, Jessica! I can be your hitch!" Stewie winked at me.

"You know what my sister has been through Stewie. That Jackson fellow, you remember me telling you about that scumbag? The carer who abused her when she was teenager?"

Stewie gravely nodded. "No one is going to take advantage of her again."

"No man will hurt her without me beating the proverbial out of them." Tom smiled and gave me a hug.

"Don't worry Jessica, one day, I can assure you that you will end up being just like Tom and Jem—totally and madly in love."

Dad finally managed to get the medics to agree that it was in my best interest that I was cared for at home. My parents were due to get training on how to use the NG tube at home. It finally looked like there was light at the end of the tunnel.

A week before the discharge was scheduled to take place,

the dietician and nutritional matron came hurrying into the room, where Dad was getting his jacket on ready to go to work.

"You can't leave with a NG tube. It's against protocol. You have to have the tube removed."

No, I can't stay here, I thought desperately. I physically couldn't manage it. If the tube was removed, I would never recover. It was as simple as that.

"Jessica's life is in danger without the tube. She's desperately ill and it's been made worse here. I'm taking her home with or without your help. I want my daughter to live."

"Look, as a dad myself, I know what he's saying," the matron said, suddenly changing his tune. "We've got to do what's best for her. Look at her, she can't survive on this ward."

"Okay." The dietician sighed, as she tried to think of an alternative. "Right, I think the only way is to get both you and your daughter to sign a form that will put the responsibility of the tube in your hands. If anything goes wrong then it is on you." She pointed at me and Dad. "If your weight hasn't improved in a month, then we will have to look at long term options."

Kip arrived with Dad in his bottle green uniform. I was moments away from freedom. Once I was pushed outside of the hospital, the cold fresh air hit my face. It was already evening time and the hospital was relatively quiet. The silence was welcomed by my sound-sensitive ears and I finally felt calm. I had broken free. I had made it out of that ward. Thank God!

"Kiddo, I didn't think I was going to be bringing you out alive from there. I'm just so relieved. We'll look after you, you're safe now." Dad choked up before turning away.

As the ambulance engine roared, the radio came on blaring out the Christmas single *The Power of Love*. As I listened to the lyrics, I thought of the love my family had for me and how they had saved my life. All the emotion I had been suppressing for weeks escaped out of me as I fully appreciated how close I had been to not surviving this ordeal. Dad hugged me and I began to uncontrollably cry with relief.

2013

CHAPTER SEVENTEEN

Mighty Oaks From Little Acorns Grow

A month had passed since I had been discharged from hospital. I managed to put on enough weight to have the naso-gastric tube removed without the need for a long-term solution. But that didn't stop Mum from measuring every ounce of input and output. She was adamant that I would never have to return to that ward again.

I was still traumatised from the whole experience. My self-confidence had taken a battering in that place and I carried with me all the comments that the staff had made both to my face and behind my back.

"We can't help you unless you help yourself."

"The tests don't show any infection markers. We don't know what's wrong with you."

The M.E. Monster relapse and the constant fear that people didn't believe how ill I was had made me feel more trapped in the same four walls than I'd ever felt before.

I had to try to focus on something to keep me going. It was my birthday in a couple of months. I was turning twenty-two and I wanted to celebrate. Birthdays always brought conflicting emotions because it was a reminder of another year that the

M.E. Monster had taken from me, but it was also a reminder of another milestone that I had not been expected to make.

Ever since I became bedbound when I was fifteen I dreamt of being able to sit in a chair for my birthday, but it hadn't been possible. I spent my sweet sixteenth lying flat in my dark hospital room, barely conscious, with balloons around the room instead of people.

Despite Dr Nice's valiant efforts to make my dream come true for my eighteenth birthday in Narnia, I had been too unwell to lift my head from the pillow. The silver lining was that the nurses managed to get me into a prom dress so I could celebrate the day with a short visit from my family.

Before I knew it, more birthdays passed, and I had spent each one being extremely poorly. When my twenty-first birthday came, and I still didn't manage to sit in a chair, I felt thoroughly depleted. It was like a never-ending nightmare. I began to question if I would ever be able to get out of this wretched bed?

I wracked my brain for an idea of what I could do, but I was distracted by my phone buzzing. It was an email from YouTube alerting me that my awareness video had now been watched by *ten thousand* people! I thought back to that film, which had been released six months ago, and I felt so proud of it. I felt like it was made a lifetime ago; the journey my life had taken since that time had involved emergencies and increased suffering.

Since then so many people from around the world had become a part of my life on social media. The Facebook page that I had set up to post about my life in one room had grown past my wildest imagination.

What could I do to surpass that? Was this going to be the year I managed to sit in a chair?

Then an idea came to me: Seven Years in the Making. I could document my struggle to sit in a chair with an awareness video like my previous one. *What if I went one step closer than that and used my social media following to give both able bodied and disabled people a chance to become part of the story?*

Now that was an idea I liked the sound of!

Having a plan made me feel mentally stronger, like there was a way forward and I had a purpose.

"What are you so happy about, Jessica?" Becky asked as she helped to wash me.

"I've got a plan and I'm going to need you to be a part of it."

"Is this your plan to escape this room? You go out on the lash in Canterbury, happen to stumble upon Orlando Bloom, who then whisks you off your feet and you go travelling?"

"That sounds like a plan for the future. To think that all the time we were in Canterbury, Orlando-bloody-Bloom's dad was going to our grandad's music concerts!"

"Precisely!" Becky laughed. "Which is why I know that I'm most certainly wrong, because I don't think Orlando would appreciate a stalker like you!"

"I'm going far better than that. I want to sit in a chair for my birthday. I'll finally use the chair that has been by my bed for seven years! I could do another awareness video to document my journey to managing it."

Becky looked down at her feet. She sighed and looked at me. "You need to make sure you're physically well enough for all of this. I mean you're still recovering from that awful admission and I can't have you get that unwell again. The image of you in that hospital bed haunts me every day." I opened my mouth to protest, but she carried on talking gently to me. "It doesn't mean I won't support you or it won't happen. Just please, don't push yourself too far."

Since my last hospital admission the community team had a different energy. My care manager had visited weekly to check how I was doing, and was assigned a new physio terrorist who was already making a massive difference to my life. It was like they had suddenly realised how immensely fragile my body was.

With this new physio terrorist I could feel there was a difference to those I had previously had within the community. I think she saw me as a challenge because she knew that anything she did movement-wise could have catastrophic effects on my body. She wasn't used to seeing patients as young as me being completely bedbound, and I think that spurred her on to try and help me.

I told her of my chair idea the next time she visited me. I needed her to understand that sitting in a chair was such an important dream that I couldn't give up on. "Right, let's break this down. I think the chair sit is a possibility but we need to think about all the components that will get you there. And that is where I see the difficulty staring back at me." The physio terrorist sighed. "So, we can plan this. You need to be able to raise your head in the bed, sit up for more than thirty seconds without collapsing, and then we have the problem of the hoist. Currently, your body is not used to gravity. You're a bit like an astronaut now."

"I suppose I would have had a better view if I was an astronaut," I joked.

"It would be even more isolating than being here. I wouldn't want to orbit in space, and be able to see the world, but not reach it."

"That is a little bit like my life is now," I said.

"Then we will give this the best shot we can to make this dream come true for you."

CHAPTER EIGHTEEN

#7yrsinthemaking

The physio terrorist broke sitting in a chair down into small chunks. There was so much to consider that it felt like an overwhelming task. The first step was to sit up in the bed for longer periods, then I had to be hoisted up into the air. My family, carers, and the whole team had to work together to make sure that I was given the best chance at being able to achieve this goal.

My blood pressure dropped every time I was hoisted up because my body struggled with gravity. The blood would pool into my feet every time I was lifted. I had fallen out of a hoist sling on two separate occasions whilst in hospital and I've hated hoists ever since, yet it was completely necessary to use one if I was ever going to manage my goal of sitting in a chair.

Through the day I spent five minutes in short increments, raising my head with the aid of my hospital bed. At first, I could only last ten seconds before an intense pain filled my head and I would begin to spin with dizziness. Exhaustion filled every part of my body before I fainted and had to be laid completely flat.

I filmed every moment documenting my journey and shared snippets on my social media. Everyone who watched the videos and updates were joining me on this journey; I was so grateful for them all.

The occupational health therapist started to work with my physio terrorist to find practical solutions to help me. She sourced a specially-made hoist sling and worked on how to make sure the recliner chair was comfortable for me. I needed cushions to protect my delicate skin, and the chair had to be able to get my feet up to prevent me from collapsing straight away. My care team and family were trained by the physio terrorist to be able to ensure the exercises continued when she wasn't there.

"Remember to look for the signs of Jessica losing consciousness. It is imperative that everyone knows what to expect."

The hoist was my biggest challenge and quickly became my arch enemy. My body was so fragile that I couldn't be lifted without fear of my bones breaking due to my osteoporosis. When I was lifted into the air, even for a few seconds, my heart would begin to race, and I would then faint. The sheer exhaustion from using the hoist was suffocating. The lights would just go out like a switch and my battery would become empty with no real warning.

The process started very slowly. Once the first step of raising my head with the bed was achieved, I had to build up the time I could do it for—this was to give me a better chance at staying in the hoist without collapsing. Becky would hold my legs up to prevent the blood pooling whilst my carer would hold my head. Although Becky was young, she was responsible for so much of my health needs and had been my young carer since she was ten.

I worked with the team for several weeks to make sure that I was able to be hoisted for the full three minutes we had estimated it would take to complete the transfer. Gradually, my tolerance of sitting up with the headrest improved and my blood pressure became more stable. The progress was painfully slow, which I found frustrating. All I could do was keep documenting all the highs and lows, from managing to sit up longer, to when it felt like it was an impossible task.

To try and help my blood pressure, I wore TED compression stockings. All my carers were trained to hoist me, but it took three people to do it. When I fainted from the exertion my body would shake uncontrollably, as the adrenaline seeped out of every cell. Then I was zapped of everything. I knew that it would take months of energy and sacrifice to achieve my goal but I couldn't wait any longer, it had to be now.

Using the online community that I had grown to love dearly, I started a campaign called #7yrsinthemaking. My plan was to release the footage I had been collecting on my birthday, no matter if I sat in the chair or not.

Dad returned to his novelty director's chair in my room, and we once again used our creativity to make a powerful video that I hoped would raise awareness to the reality that so many severely affected M.E. sufferers faced.

Social media had been a godsend to me since returning home. It made me feel less alone. I couldn't see people in person but I could still catch up with everyone. Blissy and all my other online buddies arranged to do a 'Thunderclap' on Twitter and Facebook to get the hashtag trending for my birthday.

It was a lot of pressure, but I hoped that people would really connect to the story. When I told my old friends of my plans, they couldn't even begin to imagine what it was like to want something like sitting in a chair, when they would do this constantly throughout the day without thinking, but Blissy understood. She was desperately ill with multiple chronic illnesses and she knew how important it was for me to raise awareness. In some ways it felt like it gave me purpose.

As the weeks flew by, I was progressing in the right direction. Becky was a constant support. She held on to me when it felt too much and championed my progress. My parents were more apprehensive; they knew that if I didn't manage to do the sit, I would be completely broken.

For once, the community team didn't push my body too far, despite the pressure I was putting myself under. They knew how much damage it had caused my body when it had been done previously. Even though I was desperate to fulfil this dream, I had learnt to stop if I didn't feel I could manage it. Although I told people that I wouldn't mind if I couldn't do it on the big day, the truth was I couldn't imagine how I would cope if I didn't. I was a strong-willed character that was full of hope, but there was only so much disappointment I could deal with. I just had to keep praying that 2013 would be the year.

CHAPTER NINETEEN

Happy Birthday

The day had arrived. Everything was planned to the finest detail. No matter what happened, Dad was going to make the end of the video. Becky had drawn a poster with the all-important countdown of this seven-year journey.

The TED stockings were put on, I was rolled over, so the hoist sling could be inserted, whilst Dad filmed. Before I knew it, the dream I had visualised for so long was finally happening. I held on with all my might, as the hoist moved me from my bed into the air and over to the beautiful chair. My goal was within reach.

It ran like clockwork. I closed my eyes and took in all the senses of being out of bed. The room looked completely different now I was seeing it from a different position. Once in the chair, the cake was placed in front of me, and I blew out the candles in a dreamlike state.

After thirty seconds, my head started to spin. I was quickly moved out of the chair to the bed with the hoist. I lost consciousness as my blood pressure dropped. I woke up to find myself silently shaking, as the adrenaline and exhaustion riddled my body, but I had done it! I had sat in a chair on my birthday!

An overwhelming sense of relief filled me, as Becky and my parents huddled around me and we all cried tears of joy. The wait was finally over. Something I had fought for so long to achieve had passed in a moment.

The poster that rounded up what had happened in the past seven years, was placed next to me:

7 years dreaming of this moment to happen
6 years completely bedridden
5 years hospitalised
4 years continuously so
3 years unable to move
2 years fed through a tube
1 Year Behind Dark Glasses
Still fighting severe M.E.
It's my birthday and I'm finally sitting in a chair!

I was ecstatic but there was a slight feeling of loss—how had something that took less a minute, taken seven years to achieve? *Seven whole years.*

There was not a moment longer to think about it because phase two of my plan had started. The adrenaline still pumped through my body, but it was filled with excitement as Dad uploaded the finished video to YouTube. He released a picture of me sitting in a chair and social media exploded into cheers.

Blissy began sharing it far and wide in the Facebook world. The rest of my 'online family' all started tweeting at 5pm, and Twitter went wild with hundreds of tweets celebrating the good news. In a short space of time, five thousand people had already seen the video. Both my able-bodied friends and

M.E. sufferers worked together to get the hashtag noticed by the public. I watched as the news spread and social media lit up with support for me.

At 5:30pm, the notification came through to say that #7yrsinthemaking was trending at number one in the United Kingdom! At that moment, I had achieved everything I had set out to do. Not only had I finally managed to sit in a chair, but in doing so, I had raised awareness. Even though the adrenaline had fizzled out, the satisfaction remained. The pain swamped my body, and the M.E. Monster took over.

The next morning, I painstakingly typed a message for every single person who had shared my story on my Facebook page.

There are no words that can truly define this moment. The support I have received from everybody has been completely out of this world. The only words I can manage to say through the exhaustion seem rather inadequate but thank you for making my dream come alive! I was sick, the room was spinning, but ultimately the candles were blown out in just the way I had dreamt of. Finally, I can say I did it!

The celebrations online continued throughout the week, but I had to stop and rest, as the exhaustion rendered me motionless. No amount of pain could take away from the sense of achievement that I felt. It had been the best birthday in a long time.

CHAPTER TWENTY

Kevin The Kidney Stone

I woke up with a pain in my kidney. It was a sharp pain that took my breath away. My carer rang up the doctor's surgery, and a home visit was arranged for the afternoon. I was pretty sure that nothing could be done about the pain, and I questioned if I was just causing more bother. However, I knew it was better that the doctors made this decision.

Normally, my GP would try her best to come out to me, no matter what, but she wasn't on call, so a trainee doctor came in her place. I thought I was just being overcautious by getting it checked out, because generally these sorts of pains would be considered as medical anomalies that were another bizarre M.E. symptom.

The doctor checked my pulse and listened to my stomach.

"I just can't rule out that it's not a kidney stone blocking your urethra. I think you need to go to hospital."

It came as a shock to my family as they were used to an ambulance being called as the final straw, not as a precaution. My parents were planning to go to Cambridge to sing in a choral group but had to delay, putting it down to another battle with the M.E. Monster.

It took two ambulances and four paramedics just to get me out of the house this time because Dad and Kip weren't available to help. They had no idea how difficult it was to get me out of the room, due to the angle of it. Dad and Kip were professionals as they had done it so many times! We were waiting for the extension to be made downstairs so these journeys wouldn't be quite so difficult. *Normally I'm more ill than this when I'm waiting for an ambulance,* I thought.

My parents were adamant that I wouldn't be there for long, and waved goodbye, as they finally made their way to Cambridge. I waited for the ambulance, mentally preparing myself for the incredibly loud noises, and the motion. I wondered whether Stewie would come, as I knew he was on duty. He sent me a text to say that it would be one of his mates and that he had told them to be on their best behaviour. It was questionable what 'best behaviour' meant for the lads he socialised with!

Even the smallest amount of movement caused me to be so unwell. Sometimes, I wondered whether it was worth the sheer effort it would take to get me out.

My carer frantically tried to pack my stuff and Becky kept everything together. She always kept me calm and more importantly—laughing. The commotion of having to go to hospital did not faze Becky. She was completely used to the drama of having to cancel plans to look after me.

The ambulance arrived quite quickly and I was connected to machines for an observation. They checked my heart rate, oxygen stats and temperature. Everything was okay. Other than the pain I was in and the fact that my pulse was a bit high. I had to go to the surgical assessment unit.

"Well, it's a different part of the hospital to your usual!" the paramedic said.

Soon enough, we were on the road again. There was a whole world out there that I was yet to explore. I just had my memories of it from before I had become ill. Dark glasses shielded my eyes, even though they were firmly shut. The motion of the stretcher was enough to make me physically sick, and that was without the increase in pain that I was feeling from my kidney.

We arrived at the hospital. Becky started to read me a magazine but I started to feel a bit peculiar. The healthcare assistant came in to triage me and do my observations. She put the heart rate monitor on me, as I started to feel like the lights were swimming before my eyes, due to the pulsing pain I was in. The machine started beeping as my pulse jumped to 160 and it kept increasing. My pulse kept rocketing.

165.

170.

180.

She felt my wrist and pressed the emergency assist button on the wall.

Becky threw the magazine to the side as lots of doctors and nurses came rushing into the cubicle. They tried to assess quickly where the problem was coming from. All they could see was that I was in discomfort and my pulse was now over 190 bpm. The head nurse came and took an oxygen mask off the wall.

"Okay sweetheart, I need you to stop thinking about breathing. This machine will do it for you."

They quickly realised that my bladder was in complete retention and was holding over a litre of urine in it. Whilst two doctors desperately tried to get a catheter into me, a doctor started doing arterial punches, and another tried to get a cannula in. My carer looked in dismay at the carnage, not knowing what to do. Becky held my hand tightly, as more people did different things to my body. She stroked my head and told me that it was going to be okay.

My temperature had risen from the volume of urine that was stuck, and the surgical team wondered if a kidney stone had caused me to go into retention. It was an incredibly hot day at the hospital and the unit was stifling.

I looked up at Becky, as her grip on my hand loosened significantly. She was starting to sway and before I had a moment to call out, the nurses escorted her out of the room before she fainted.

It transpired that in all the drama, she hadn't remembered to have a drink or any food since breakfast. The nurses started pumping her with ice cream and custard creams to bring up her blood sugar. After what seemed like an age, they managed to pierce my bladder with a catheter, and it started to release some of the huge amount of fluid that was stuck. My pulse dropped to 150 bpm and the atmosphere started to get a lot easier. The oxygen continued to be pumped through a mask, which was like a fan being blown into my face.

Once the doctors were happy that I was stable, they sent me for an emergency CT scan that showed I had a kidney stone blocking my urethra. Thankfully, it didn't look like it was a big one but I needed to be admitted on to a ward with some IV antibiotics and morphine to flush it out.

"That is one way to skip triage, Jessica," Becky said, as she re-joined me.

My parents returned from Cambridge, walked into the surgical assessment and their mouths dropped open. I was breathing into an oxygen mask, with machines connected to me, checking my observations.

"Well you've certainly missed a lot. The proverbial hits the fan when you aren't here!" Becky said.

After a handover, I was moved to another surgical ward, where I was put under more observations and IV medications. It seemed the worst of it was over but then I suddenly started to be violently sick with a raging temperature. The doctors had been debating whether I would need to have an emergency operation to put a stent into my kidney. They were convinced that my problems passing urine, and the granules in the samples, meant the stone was still stuck there.

Someone stayed with me throughout the day, as I was dependent on others. I laid completely still, with beads of sweat appearing on my forehead. I couldn't leave the bed, even with a hoist, because the medical emergency had caused my body to crash. The M.E. Monster was tormenting me, as the inevitable setback took over.

How was it possible that only twenty-four hours ago I was laughing and joking with Becky? A week ago, I was being hoisted into a chair?

I had just started to increase the length of time I was able to sit. I had just managed to spend a minute out of the bed and now the M.E. Monster had humiliated me. I didn't even have the energy to turn my head to reach the vomit bowl before I was sick.

The hospital bay was horrendously loud and all the sounds of the ward made me wince with pain. The woman who was opposite me had lost her limbs due to smoking when she was younger. As Mum chatted to her, she said how desperately she wanted to show other people about what smoking can really do. My carer moved uncomfortably from side to side, as she tried to stop herself from needing another smoke.

I decided that this wretched kidney stone needed to have a name. If it was going to cause so much trouble, then I needed to be on first name terms with it. It reminded me of a stroppy teenager, so I went with Kevin, from the movie *Kevin and Perry Go Large*.

As the weekend passed on, my health continued to deteriorate, and the doctors agreed that I needed to be operated on as soon as possible. Not long after the decision was made, my bed was pushed down to theatre. All I could think about was an episode of the TV show *Casualty*, where the patient had died on the operating table. I just hoped that I would survive.

CHAPTER TWENTY-ONE

HDU

A mask was placed over my face and they started injecting something into my cannula. It was all very clinical; they didn't talk as they were so focused. As I looked at the anaesthetist, I decided that the reason they had a rubbish bedside manner was because they were used to the patients being asleep. I felt more ill-at-ease because no one could understand when I was trying to say something, or when I needed help. I dreaded waking up in the middle of the operation or needing something. The doctors barely knew of the disease, as hospitals were not normal surroundings for M.E. patients to be found in.

In seconds, I was out like a light and the operation took place. I woke up to what felt like just a few moments later, when it was in fact a good few hours later. It was excruciatingly painful in my kidney area. Kevin was continuing to cause a lot of problems. No one had warned me that the stent would be just as painful as having Kevin lurking in the background.

As they tried to rouse me, I could feel the tube that had kept me safe through the operation being tugged, but I was too drowsy to stir. The surgeons tried to wake me up more and found that my observations were a little low. I had always been difficult to wake from surgery; anaesthetic used to knock me for six. When I did wake up, there was a sharp stabbing pain in my side.

Finally, I was taken back to the ward, where they kept me going with IV fluids and antibiotics. I still had a raging temperature and felt very rough from the surgery. The M.E. Monster caused me to have very extreme reactions to surgery. My body seemed to react in a bad way to everything that was thrown at it.

I remained in hospital for the next few days, whilst the medics tended to my fever. One of the nurses was an old family friend, Sarah, who had started her nursing when I became unwell. Thank goodness she was there. She kept a firm eye on me and made sure that I was looked after to the best of her ability. When the doctors said that I could go home, she insisted that I needed to stay a little while longer, until my fever was more under control. She acted as a lifeline to me.

It was so hot in the hospital that I had to keep hydrated with ice lollies and a fan on me. Mum struggles with the heat, so she spent all her time making sure me and all the other patients were as comfortable as possible. To go home, I had to be able to pee and fully empty my bladder. At first I was still being monitored with a catheter in situ—that caused more problems than it was worth. Some of the granules from Kevin the Kidney Stone were stuck in the tubes of the catheter. The urine started to build up and it was agonisingly painful.

"Help me!" I yelled as Sarah passed me.

By this time, my tummy was incredibly swollen with the amount of urine that was stuck in my bladder. Yet the catheter was not flowing. I couldn't focus on anything else and my body shook uncontrollably as I waited for help.

Please take it out. Take the catheter out. It's hurting so much!" I screamed as Sarah came up to my bed.

Sarah tried to flush it, but it made no difference. She decided to take the catheter out. As soon as it was removed, I filled two bedpans in quick succession. She did a bladder scan that confirmed my bladder was now empty, which meant I was one step closer to home.

Once I was finally discharged, Dad arranged for him and Kip to take me home.

Kip entered with a massive grin on his face. "Jessica! It's been a while, young lady! And you're going to leave before food time? What are you doing to me girl?"

Missing the hospital cuisine was one of my best tricks because the food was disgusting. I would much rather wait and have something at home. My side was still very sore because the stent was keeping the urethra open a lot further than it would normally. I winced in pain with every movement, and it was even more painful when I had to empty my bladder.

A week after the ordeal had begun, I was on my way home. I realised quite how close it had been to life turning out very differently. In six weeks I would have to return to hospital to have another operation, to remove the stent and Kevin the Kidney Stone. At first I didn't really understand why they couldn't have just removed bloody Kevin when they put the stent in, but I was informed that my urethra tube wasn't big enough and had to be stretched by the stent first. It was imperative that I rested and took one day at a time.

Six weeks passed by quickly and I was in so much pain that the surgery couldn't come soon enough. I went into hospital for the pre-op assessment and the anaesthetist said that she wanted me to have a bed on the High Dependency Unit (HDU) after surgery due to my complex medical history.

Everything was thoroughly planned; I was looking forward to finally getting rid of Kevin the Kidney Stone that had rocked my life. I came into the unit to be observed. Once the bed was confirmed I was taken through to theatre. It was much more relaxed than the previous surgery, as it wasn't an emergency, so my family were there to see me before and after the operation.

Again, there were problems with waking me up from the surgery. I was incredibly drowsy. The poor anaesthetist urgently started calling my name. "Why isn't she waking up yet?"

She started doing a sternal rub but I couldn't move to say I was there. It felt oddly like an out of body experience, I could hear the surgeons talking, but I couldn't communicate back.

After a long time, I was wheeled into recovery and left there for a while, until they could take me up to HDU. I had an oxygen machine attached to me through nasal tubes to help me breathe. Despite feeling incredibly rough, I was so grateful to be able to breathe for myself. I would never take that for granted.

The pain was still there but was a lot better than it had been. Once I had been wheeled up to HDU, I was determined to get home as quickly as possible. Kevin had caused enough problems as it was. I needed to recover.

The next day, the doctors said if I could manage a meal, I could be discharged. Thankfully, I was able to. As I waited for the transport to come and take me home, I was aware of just how fortunate I had been in my near-death experience. It was only then that I fully comprehended that the trainee GP, who came to my house seven weeks prior, had saved my life. If it had been my GP who had come to me on that fateful day, would she have sent me into hospital as quickly as the trainee had? I knew that because I downplayed the pain I was in, my GP would have opted to let me stay at home, rather than go through the trauma of hospital, and if that had happened, it would've been a very different ending.

It made me think that maybe God was just playing it out right, so everything fell into place and I ended up in the hospital at just the right time, when the right people were there to help me.

CHAPTER TWENTY-TWO

Eight Years And Counting

A new M.E. charity got in touch with me after hearing my story and offered to arrange a grant for me to be able to return to Narnia to recuperate from the horrors of the past two months. I couldn't believe my luck!

When I arrived at Narnia, everything felt better. Dr Nice came and knelt by my bed, held my hand and reassured me that everything was going to be okay. He had saved my life on multiple occasions, so I trusted him.

"You've been through such a terrible ordeal, but you survived because that's what you're good at doing. In all the moments that I've been worried about whether you were going to pull through, I've remembered to believe in you because you—" He pointed gently at me with one hand whilst holding my hand with his other. "Are one hell of a fighter."

As I came to terms with the scary truth of what had happened to me, I really needed that solace. To see someone who believed in me implicitly, gave me the reassurance that I needed. It was okay to be scared. I was not beaten, not yet, not ever. I felt so much gratitude as familiar people nursed me back to health.

Narnia was the perfect place for me to rest and recuperate. I desperately needed that. I felt relieved because I knew I was in the safe hands of a medical team led by Dr Nice, who understood the complexities of M.E. far better than anyone else. The past few months had been a rather unpleasant rollercoaster, and I was being forced to come to terms with my own mortality after *that* surgical experience.

The M.E. Monster had been far from kind to me since Kevin the Kidney Stone had been removed. It had hit me with electrical and muscular pain all over my body, rather than the localised spot where Kevin had been. The fatigue felt like I had been hit head on with a double-decker bus that was full to the brim with exhaustion.

The payback from the operation meant that I hadn't been able to contemplate being hoisted from my bed to the chair again. My baseline was currently back to hardly having the energy to move my body for myself and needing to use the controls for the bed to lift my head up.

Dr Nice kept reminding me of how far I had come since he first met me. "You've been on such an incredible journey, Jessica. I know this is tough, you've suffered so much due to this blasted Monster. But just like the phoenix in your favourite book series *Harry Potter,* you will rise again."

He always knew how to make me smile. I told him about Seven Years in the Making, on the off chance that he hadn't watched the YouTube video yet, and he was impressed. The success of that momentous achievement on my birthday had given me the confidence to keep going forward. So much of my life had been dictated by the Monster that I didn't really know what I could do for myself anymore.

Dr Nice adjusted my pain relief to make me more comfortable, with the hope that it would enable me to benefit from the physio terrorist. When she came around, she asked me what I would like to work towards from her visits.

My current limitations meant that there was very little chance that I would be able to get out of bed into my specialised chair. That was clear. *What else would I like to do?* I pondered on my very long bucket list of goals I would love to manage one day. I thought of the rush of endorphins that I got every time I managed to sit in a chair and see the world the right way up. When I did that first sit, it had made me feel like I was becoming alive again, after years of only being able to exist and survive every torturous moment of this disease. Yes, that is what I wanted to work towards; being able to sit on the edge of the bed with assistance.

The physio terrorist and I spoke about how to break down my goal into sizeable chunks. The first of which was working out how the hell I could get my body to turn over on my own. Since being unwell I had not been able to move around by myself. As I didn't have the muscle to move anymore, my body felt like a weight that couldn't be lifted.

To begin with we started working on the mechanics of getting my muscles to receive the neurological pathways that my brain sent, to tell them to move independently. It had been such a long time since I had moved independently that they didn't know how to work on their own.

The first mission was to be able to roll on to my side on my own, which currently took two people to do it. This would give my body the start that it needed to get used to the movement. The simple pleasure of just being able to move on to my side when I was uncomfortable couldn't be under-estimated.

"Right Jessica, we're going to try by getting you to clench your glutes," the physio terrorist said. She could see me trying but my muscles protested. "I can see a twitch there! Well done! Your body is going to feel a lot heavier but you're doing great. Okay, now rest. Just try doing that in repetitions a few times a day. I want to turn on those brain signals."

The next time I saw her, we tried again and even in that short space of time, my glutes seemed to be twitching more and trying to move by themselves.

"Everything is a process. We must work with your body and go at its pace. It's important that we don't force your body to exercise when you're physically struggling," she explained.

I continued to work on the mechanics of my muscles. Slowly but surely, I was able to move independently. Once I was able to move my glutes, I had to work on my core muscles, with the hope that I could start to heave my body over on to its side. It was amazing to witness how quickly my body remembered movements that it had last done many years ago. The imprints of moving on to my side had been ingrained into me since I was a baby. Naturally, my muscles realised that I was trying to do something I had done millions of times before. It was as if I was giving myself a spring clean and wiping the dust off the part of my brain which controlled movement.

Once my muscles were reacting, the carers helped me to try to move on my side. The physio terrorist came up with different techniques to enhance my body's capabilities.

"You know what? I think that this technique will really work. All you need to do is imagine that you're rolling on to your side. Think about what each muscle has to do and imagine them working perfectly." She grinned as I looked at her quizzically. "This is what athletes do all the time. You know at the start of a race; they look like they're in the zone? That is them running the race before they have physically run it. I promise you! Basically, your body doesn't understand a lie, so if you think you're doing it, you will go through all the physical processes as if it were actually happening."

It sounded odd and I was dubious as to whether it would work. As I continued to work on it, I found that the cognitive activity of the neurological pathways telling my body to move was more exhausting than the physical movement itself.

When my physio terrorist arrived for my last session at Narnia she was convinced that I would roll over. The carer filmed me as I put into practice all that she had taught me; I thought about the signals reaching my core muscles and my glutes, then I focused on using the neurological signal to get them to heave my body onto its side. The muscles in my trunk took the lead and I started to move my bottom to push my body over. Everything had to work in perfect harmony. As my body successfully turned onto my side relief washed over me.

The nurse and physio terrorist clapped their hands to their mouth in delight. They had worked with me through times when I was unable to eat, speak or even wiggle a finger. Now, they were witnessing my body waking up again after such a long time. After everything that I had been through in the past three months, I felt so proud of myself.

Dr Nice had quietly come into my room and watched me do my new trick. "Jessica, you are so resilient. You could've been beaten by all that you've been through, but instead you show that act of defiance of not letting these experiences mould who you are. You've definitely got this! We will be having our boxing match in no time! Are you still going to be in the blue corner?"

Since he'd first met me all those years ago, he'd been convinced that one day we'd have a boxing match. It wasn't because I was particularly interested in boxing but when my arms had been in big splints by my side, they looked like I was wearing boxing gloves. Dr Nice always joked that one day we'd have a boxing match where I would get my own back for the years of him accidently calling me Jess, instead of Jessica.

"Yep, I will be in the blue corner and I think I will definitely succeed!"

"I've no doubt you will!" he laughed.

CHAPTER TWENTY-THREE

Mind Control

Once I returned home, I had to navigate myself through the unforgiving payback that the M.E. Monster thwarted me with. The level of fatigue I felt would often cause me to lose my speech and prevent me from being able to move. All I could do was wait patiently for the flare-up to pass.

After a month of adjusting to being back at home in my world of one room, I started to feel well enough to slowly increase my functions. I had enough energy to hold some conversations and I even managed to start moving my body again.

I was desperate to be able to sit back in my chair like before Kevin the Kidney Stone disrupted my life, so I began to use the control of the bed to raise my head. I gently practised being able to coax my body into starting to roll over again on my own. It started with doing the same mind technique that the physio terrorist at Narnia had taught me, to make my body feel like it had already managed to do it.

Then it finally happened: my body managed with huge effort to heave me on to my side. A thought popped into my head as I showed Becky and Mum my new party trick from my stay in Narnia. *What would happen if I tried to lift my head off the pillow too?*

I felt a sudden surge of adrenaline, as I tried to roll on to my side and then, just like that, I pushed on to my forearm and lifted my head off the pillow for the first time, with relative ease. It was as if my body remembered what it was meant to do, I didn't even need to give it much thought.

From that moment, I wanted to shout from the rooftops about what I achieved. I continued to practise my fine motor skills when I felt well enough, to try and test the water on what else could be possible for my body to do. It had taken me eight years to be able to roll over on my side on my own. My fortune seemed to be changing, and although it had taken over a third of my lifespan, I was convinced that muscle memory was going to be the key to my progress.

I wanted to be careful about the exercises because I suffered terribly in the past, at the hands of the harmful therapy called Graded Exercise, which I was forced into doing in hospital. I remembered the horror so clearly, when my physio terrorist as teenager dictated that the headrest was raised every day without fail. She demanded that the angle it was put up to was increased by thirty percent every three days, despite my sobs of pain. It had been disastrous for my body and took many years to recover from.

I would only attempt to roll over when I felt strong enough to do it. If I felt too unwell, I would stop. Every time I managed to roll over, I was reminded of the children's nursery rhyme *Ten in a Bed.* The tune played over in my head.

There were ten in the bed and the little one said, "Roll over," so we all rolled over, and one fell out!

Being able to roll over was such a normal occurrence for people who weren't disabled. Although my friends were so excited for me when I told them what I could do, they couldn't begin to fathom how it felt to rejoice in something that was such a small part of their day. They had never had to think about it when they rolled over. Instead, they would do it half asleep to turn the alarm off in the morning before work. To them, there was nothing magical about getting up for work in the mornings. For me, it was my greatest dream. Now that I had successfully managed to lift my head from the pillow, I was convinced that sitting on the edge of the bed with assistance was a possibility.

I woke up one morning feeling like my battery, which always had low energy, was a bit fuller than I was used to. When my carer came to my bed to help me I set up my camera on the bedside table and asked her to support my trunk. She looked quizzically at me as I smiled back at her. She nervously put her hands on my torso. "What are you up to Jessica?"

My emergency hospital admission with Kevin had terrified her, due to the rate I had deteriorated in her care. She had been adamant ever since that I didn't push my body.

I set my eyes on the camera that was recording on selfie mode and began to attempt to get my body to move. My carer tentatively looked at me, as she watched my body begin to tremor.

"Are you sure you're ready for this? I don't even really know what you're about to do. . . please. . . please be careful."

My body moved as I asked it to and my carer's face turned from being alarmed to joy as she watched me move more freely. I rolled over and began to lift my full torso through my forearm. I shook uncontrollably but I managed to get a glimpse of the world the right way up. For a fleeting moment, I looked into the camera where my face was staring back at me in selfie mode.

My carer gasped and her eyes filled with tears. She held on to my shoulders to support me as she cheered.

"Jesus, Mary and Joseph and all the saints! Look at you!"

Sitting up, I could see a shadow of Gran in my reflection in the selfie mode of the camera. I only stayed upright for a few seconds, but it had a lasting effect on me. Although Gran was not there physically, she lived on through my family. It reminded me of the *Lion King* and I tried to imagine Rafiki telling me, "She lives in you."

Becky and I had always looked similar to Gran, but it was only now, seeing myself upright, that I could process the resemblance. It had been so long since I had last seen myself that I didn't recognise the reflection. I looked completely different to the photo hanging on the wall of my room, of the last time I sat up. As I looked at that photo, I felt like I was looking at entirely different person. Not only was my hair considerably shorter, but my facial structure had changed too.

I was left with an odd cacophony of emotions as I stared at the video that I had just recorded. Despite being incredibly happy that I managed another big goal I had been working towards, I felt disconnected from the video of the stranger looking back at me. My identity was lost. All I could see was what the M.E. Monster had left behind, and it wasn't a pretty sight.

CHAPTER TWENTY-FOUR

Christmas Catheters

Tom came to visit just before he was due to fly out with Jem on a trip to Paris. We were all excited to see him as he rarely managed to make the trip from Basingstoke to Kent. He came into my room and whispered in my ear, "Can you keep a secret?"

"Yeah, of course I can!"

He put his hand into his pocket and brought out a ring box. As soon as I saw the diamond sparkle, my eyes lit up. I was going to have a sister-in-law!

"I've told her we're going to Paris for the Christmas market. I'm going to ask her to marry me, but keep it quiet." He winked and left the room.

Tom rang a few days later and confirmed that Jem had said yes! Everyone was ecstatic at the thought of having a new JT in the family.

"I remember you saying you wanted me to wait to get married until you were well enough to go to it. Well, we're going to be waiting two years, so get on to it, sis."

Challenge accepted, I thought.

On Christmas Eve I started to systematically work out the

goals I would need to achieve to get to the wedding, so I could discuss it with the medical team after they came back from leave. However, I started to feel really unwell. My temperature rose, and my tummy started to hurt.

The doctor was called as I couldn't pass urine. I grew paler and paler and the pain in my bladder was excruciating.

Not another kidney stone, I thought desperately.

After the doctor came and confirmed that my bladder was in retention, the ambulance was called. Becky came in with a Santa hat. She put one on my head before she laid on the bed next to me.

"Your body always chooses a special occasion or a weekend in which to mess around!" she said. "Yes, I remember the appendicitis, Easter, the Christmases, birthdays and weekends spent holding my head up with my hand, trying not to fall asleep at some godforsaken hour."

I snorted with laughter, as she continued with her monologue on how my body seemed to dislike important family occasions. Now, she was describing the unbearable hunger she had felt on all of those hospital times and the indecency of closing the hospital shop at night, relying solely on vending machines.

"Do you remember that time when you were being sick and couldn't eat?"

"Which time was that? There have been a few!"

"The cornflakes incident." She shuddered and heaved slightly. "I remember it like it was yesterday. You were stuck in bed, unable to eat anything and it had taken most of the night to get you moved to an acute medical ward. We were nowhere near the shop to get some food. The breakfast trolley came around in the morning and I explained to the lady that you weren't able to eat anything. She was appalled that she would leave a cubicle without leaving something, so she let me have some on your behalf. I eyed up the cornflakes. They looked so good. The lady poured some out and my tummy started gurgling, then she poured a disproportionate amount of milk all over them before I could tell her that I didn't want milk. There is nothing I hate more than cereal with milk!"

I laughed so much that it hurt my swollen bladder. I winced. Becky had always been such an eccentric character who had been forced to grow up before Mother Nature was ready, due to the strains of having a seriously unwell sister. She was so mature for an eighteen year old.

Becky looked at me. "The poor cornflakes were drowning in milk—full fat milk, might I add—just to make it even more sickly. The problem was I felt bad for—"

"What the cornflakes?" I joked.

"Jessica, this scarred me for life. Don't laugh at my disposition." She winked at me. "I felt bad for the lady who would come back to see I hadn't touched it, so I tried to eat them and gagged every time. They were ruined. There are not many things I believe in after all we've been through but karma, my friend, is one of them. It was a travesty!"

There was a knock at the door, then the chatter of people, marking the arrival of the ambulance.

Becky jumped up quickly, fumbling in her bag, "Wait! If we're going to hospital and have to go out on Christmas Eve then we bring Christmas to hospital. That means you need a picture with your Santa hat. I will update The World of One Room Page with a picture and insert 'Merry Bloody Christmas.'"

The voices got louder and started to come up the stairs.

Becky reverted to her shy self, as she gathered all my bits for an overnight bag. Before long, I had made the long journey over the top of bannister—we were still waiting for the plans of the extension to be finalised.

My stomach was heavily bloated. The M.E. Monster screamed and hissed inside at the noises and motion, making me whimper at the pain I was in. I breathed in the Entonox, which numbed my senses. As we arrived at the local hospital, all the paramedics were out in full force asking after Dad and Tom. Becky rolled her eyes as Dad got into another conversation with someone else he knew.

As soon as I was triaged, I was moved to an acute ward.

"This had better not end the same way as the cornflakes incident!" Becky whispered into my ear.

I laughed through the pulsing pain. It had become apparent that I was going to need a catheter fitted to drain the urine. It was safe to say I was hesitant, but I was sure it couldn't be that bad.

First, a nurse came in and prepared me for the worse. Becky held my hand. Dad left to give me some dignity. Blimey, it is such an undignified position to be in. She put some jelly on the end of the catheter and the pain was extreme. *Was this how it was meant to feel? Or had it gone wrong?*

"Oh, I'm sorry, it has missed somehow," the nurse said. "Please can we try again?"

She tried again and again and again. My yells could be heard for the entire ward to hear. I could almost feel my bladder palpating in the agony.

Dad tried to come in when the frazzled nurse came rushing out.

"Alright sweetheart, I'm so sorry. I'll get some help."

I laid there with tears in my eyes.

"Oh honey, it sounds so painful. I'm sure they must be able to get it in next time," Dad said just as a doctor came in.

"I hear we have catheter problems here. Would you mind if I had a go, Jessica?" he asked.

I nodded unceremoniously. Now I knew what it felt like to have a tube pushed into areas a tube should not go. It was the same story—he tried again and again. By which time, I had given up on this being a quick and easy process.

"I don't understand, it's going in somewhere," the bewildered male doctor said before exiting whilst making excuses that he was going to find a senior doctor.

"Hasn't mastered female anatomy, clearly," Becky whispered. "Honestly, I don't know how you're doing it. It's making me sweat with the sheer idea of it. Seriously, you're doing so well. It's okay we're going to make it into a damn good Christmas after this."

Another doctor came in shortly after. "Hello Jessica, I hear the nurses and the previous doctor are having some problems putting in the catheter? We really need to get it in, so would you mind if I gave it a go?"

I shook my head but this time the pain was so intense that I was squeezing Becky's hand as I cried out.

He missed.

It was torturous as they kept trying and I was beginning to bleed. Again and again. Screams weren't enough to contain the agony that my insides were going through. How could so many people be missing? He tried again with no success. This was now the twelfth attempt.

"How can they piss it up so much? No pun intended," Becky said in disbelief. "You must have a seriously messed up system or there is something wrong with what they learnt at medical school."

The registrar came in a few minutes later. It had now been over an hour to get a catheter in. The usual spiel came, "Hi Jessica, I'm the registrar for the ward so I'm hoping I will be able to get this blasted catheter in. Is that okay?"

I nodded. By now the pain from the M.E., the noises, the lights, the adrenaline that was keeping me going was starting to melt away. All my M.E. symptoms were starting to flare up, my bladder felt like it was being pulverised as the fluid retained more and went back up to my kidneys. I was counting on him. Yet again, he could not get the tube into the right place. He tried three times.

"You're doing so well love," Becky whispered, as she stroked my head and held on to my hand.

"Okay, Jessica, I'm so sorry but I'm failing here so I'm going to call it a day and page the consultant." He hurried off.

"Still no luck?" Dad called through the curtains.

"No," Becky said exasperated. "What a start to Christmas this is."

The consultant, the registrar, two junior doctors and a nurse came in my cubicle. My private parts had become an exhibition!

"Listen Jessica, I'm going to give this one attempt and hopefully we shall get this bladder draining. I'm sorry there's been so much hassle. I should have been called sooner," the consultant urologist noted my Christmas attire. "At least you're ready for Christmas."

I secretly thought that I wasn't quite ready, and couldn't care less about Christmas, unless he could get the catheter in. The nurse poured some numbing gel over the trauma spot, and I held my breath, whilst Becky squeezed my hand and he went for me with the tube and got it in straight away. Hallelujah! I could immediately start to feel the pressure start to ease slightly on my bloated bladder. Even the consultant let out a sigh of satisfaction.

"We need to keep you in overnight then we will send you home tomorrow with the catheter. It will need to be kept in for a week and the district nurses can remove it. Sound like a plan?" He spoke quickly but calmly.

"Yes. . . it. . . does," I wearily emphasised each word.

The catheter was far from comfortable but hopefully it would just do its bloody job and we could be done with it.

Once all the medical staff had left the room, Becky sighed. "Crikey JT, I don't know how you do it, I really don't. That took over an hour and half of constantly trying to get a tube up you. I think I know the female anatomy better than them."

With that, she began to update my new Facebook page, The World of One Room. She need add no extra drama to the worst Christmas Eve so far.

It had taken so long to secure the catheter that visiting time was well and truly over. Becky lingered by the bed, until a nurse came over and said that she had to go. Dad beckoned her over to him and gave her a hug.

"We'll see you tomorrow," Dad said. "Remember to keep that Santa hat on, and you never know, Father Christmas may fix you up with a much-needed drink when you get home."

"Don't do anything I wouldn't, sis." Becky quipped, as she waved goodbye.

Then they left and I was on my own. I watched my phone as it turned to midnight, and I wished myself a happy Christmas, before trying to get some sleep.

CHAPTER TWENTY-FIVE

The Cunning Plan

In the early morning, I awoke to a pain in the cannula in my hand. A nurse stood quietly over me, as she slowly pushed medication into me. There was a commotion in one of the other cubicles, which involved a lot of screaming, so I gave up on the idea of sleep and instead decided to busy myself on my phone.

To my surprise, there were a huge number of messages from Blissy and many others from my social media that weren't just saying the usual 'Merry Christmas.' Instead, I had been forwarded a link to a national newspaper article that had shared my story.

"Jessica, this is going to make such a difference! And on Christmas Day! You must get home darling one, your Christmas pressies are awaiting you." Blissy had written in a message to me.

The nurses had also checked the newspaper. It was amazing, finally people were talking about severe M.E. and they were interested in finding out more. For a moment, it was as if a light had been shone on to my life, which had been hidden for a long time.

A nurse came round to tell me that I had a visitor. I couldn't imagine who would come to see me on Christmas Day, but then I saw Stewie pop around the corner with a Santa hat and a tacky Christmas jumper.

"When will you learn that Christmas and hospital should not be mixed in the same sentence?" He gave me a gentle hug. "You'd better get well enough to go home, because I don't appreciate having to come into this place on my only day off in the festive period!"

I couldn't help but grin.

After a few hours, the doctors came around and said that I could go home with a catheter in situ. The district nurses would have to come and check on me every day until they could remove it.

Once I finally made the trip home in the ambulance, my body crashed hard. My phone was continuously buzzing, as more people found the article online. However, for now, all goals for the wedding were put on hold until the New Year, as finally the M.E. Monster took over and I fell into a dazed rest. An eventful Christmas seemed to be a Taylor tradition that we needed to stop.

As soon as the catheter was removed two weeks later by the district nurse, I was hit by a kidney infection that knocked me for six. The M.E. Monster made sure I suffered greatly when my body was ill. I stayed hidden in my room, where I hibernated. The Monster caused my health to fluctuate significantly all the time, which was incredibly frustrating.

Every time I flicked on to social media, I could see pictures of all my friends I had been to school with, travelling the world. I had to find a way of managing my own limitations without getting jealous of what they were able to do. The power of my imagination helped to comfort me when I was feeling trapped within my own surroundings.

I dreamt of becoming more mobile and independent. I wanted to be able to do more firsts. Ever since I sat in a chair, I had been desperate to feel that euphoria again. I had been ill in bed for so long that I had forgotten what it was like to be well.

I kept myself occupied by volunteering for the charity that I had founded in 2010 called Share a Star. I designed unique holding stars for seriously unwell children and teenagers, depending on what their interests were. It had come from the idea that society calls those people that we look up to stars— whether that be film stars, pop stars or sports stars—but what about those who were fighting for their lives? In my eyes, they were stars too.

I had been thinking of trying to do some sort of fundraising for Share a Star, so the charity could continue to provide support for the families we helped.

"Becky, what can I do to help?" I said one afternoon when she was sat on my bed. Becky went quiet as she thought hard. "What about a bed push? Think about it, you could lie in the bed and Dad could push you around. . . wait a moment—" Her eyes lit up with excitement. "A bed push around Bluewater shopping centre! I mean just think back to when you were in hospital in 2006 and Psycho Woman was trying to have you put into a locked ward in London. She was determined that you were clinically depressed and your illness was all in your head. Your diary entry about wanting to go shopping at Bluewater was the only thing that made her see sense."

"You really do have the best ideas."

"The light and the noise would be a challenge for you. In a sense, going around a shopping centre is like running a marathon for you."

"I think it's time to go full circle and go shopping in Bluewater." I grinned.

My carer continued to do passive exercises to mobilise my joints and keep the range of movement. I began to feel a bit better with the antibiotics. Over time, we built up so I could join in with gentle Pilates exercises when I felt able to.

"It's your birthday in a few months, are you planning any form of celebration or goal?" my carer asked.

"Not really, I mean, I haven't even thought of it."

"I've never known you not to come up with something you want to do to mark your birthday, like when you did Seven Years in the Making."

She helped me sit up in the bed and I looked down at my legs. They seemed to go on forever.

I was in the middle of puberty when I became bed bound, not only had I continued to grow, but my bones had prematurely aged due to the lack of gravity. Since my diagnosis of severe osteoporosis in 2010, the medics had said that I would never stand or walk again. There was a vague hope that they would be able to get me into a chair. I thought about the fact I had often managed to do far more than the doctors had thought would be possible. Was this another one of those moments?

An idea hit me. *What if I did focus on being able to stand up again?* I had the right support, the right team with me. The extension was due to be completed this year, so I would finally be in an accessible room. As there was nowhere else suitable, the council had been forced to fund me staying at Narnia for the duration of the build.

Surely this was a sign? I thought.

A name hit me like a bolt of lightning. It could be called Long Way Up and I could document my journey to standing up. I looked again at my legs. It was incredible to think that if I did manage to stand up, it would be the first time that I would have seen the world from that height. What with that idea and the bed push, I could see that this was going to be a defining year for me.

2014

CHAPTER TWENTY-SIX

Stand Tall, Stand Proud

When my physio terrorist next visited, I explained my plan to her. She looked at my range of movements to assess how I was managing since my eventful Christmas.

"If we can do it we'll have to break it down into stages. The first thing we need to look at is your blood pressure, because without an improvement in that, we won't get anywhere."

"How can I do that?"

"You need to be able to have your feet on the ground without the blood pooling in them. I think we can give it a go."

She lowered the height of the bed and assisted me as I sat up. She moved my legs over the edge of the bed and for the first time since I was fifteen years old, I felt the ground. A smile appeared on my face as I felt the surreal sensation of weight going through my feet. For a few seconds I sat still, completely overwhelmed at being able to feel gravity in my body. It didn't take long before my blood pressure dropped and I started to feel lightheaded as the blood pooled down into my feet. My body became floppy and I could hear the physio terrorist calling my name. It felt distant and then it went dark as I collapsed.

When I came to, I was staring at the ceiling with my legs

elevated. My carer sat by my side, but I couldn't see the physio terrorist. A wave of exhaustion washed over me and I felt physically sick. As I tried to move my body, the M.E. Monster snarled at me. It felt like every cell in my body was screaming at me. Then it went dark and I was out again.

"Jessica, can you hear me?" my carer whispered, as she softly stroked my face.

I desperately tried to respond but the room was swaying and I felt like the M.E. Monster was suffocating me. There had to be another way I could communicate. My eyes searched my bedside table for anything. All I could see was my iPod Touch, which was out of reach.

I managed to utter the word "iPod" which she held in front of me so I could try to type out my message. My finger shook with the effort it took to move it across the screen. My arm felt so heavy that my carer had to support it. I spent an inordinate amount of time typing seven words. It was demoralising to be so vulnerable and unwell after a small change. Tears erupted down my carer's face, as she read the message that I had typed out.

Please help me. I just want to get better.

For the next few days, I had to let my body fully recover, until we found a new plan. I thought of the time that my friend had once said that it was easy to get ill, the getting better was hard. She had never been so right. It felt like I was climbing a mountain, but I couldn't see which way I was going because of the fog.

The physio terrorist returned a week later to assess me. "Nice to see you conscious, Jessica!"

I smiled weakly—it had been a tough payback that I was still struggling a week later.

"So, it's obvious that was too much for your fragile body, so we need to slow down."

"How do we slow down when that was the first step?" I groaned.

"We have your uber-cool bed, which is not just *any* bed, it's a hospital bed. They do a hell of a lot more than your average bed—they move." She took the control from the bed rail and started to put her fingers on the different buttons. "I just can't remember which one is which, even though I work with them every day."

At first, she raised the headrest up and shook her head before bring it back down. Then she put in a knee break and my legs started to elevate.

"Dammit!" she tutted before she pressed the final button, and the whole bed started to point downwards.

I could immediately feel the sensation of blood going into my legs and I was still conscious after five minutes. Hope ignited in my tummy once again and I grinned.

"How do you feel?"

"I'm okay. I'm actually okay!"

"Let's stop right there." She looked at my puzzled face. "We're *not* pushing it too far this time. You've got to build it up. Homework for this session is to try doing a couple of minutes every day when you feel up to it. Remember, slow and steady wins the race."

Over the next couple of weeks, I started to use the bed controls more. I started with just tilting the whole bed at different periods of the day and then I started to lift my headrest up as well to mimic the position that I would be in if I was sitting on the edge of the bed with my feet down.

The next task was getting my feet to be able to push down on the wooden end of the bed to try and imitate what the floor felt like for my feet. My feet were so delicate from not being able to stand up and walk that it hurt to put weight through them for more than a couple of seconds. My carer did passive exercises on my legs and I also tried to resist the movement to try and build some more strength in them. The possibility of being able to stand up fuelled my determination.

Whenever I wasn't experimenting with the controls of the bed or having passive exercises done to me, I laid flat in my bed to try and rest. I would imagine my one room to be on the top of the tranquil Bluebell Hill, where I could just lie for ages looking at the trees as they danced a slow waltz with the wind and the sun touched the back of my head. I could watch as the birds argued with one another in the bushes. I could see for miles. This visualisation helped me to relax a little bit more through the pain.

After a month of persistence, I slowly built up to try and sit with my feet on the ground again. It was physically exhausting and every time my body would begin to shake uncontrollably through the exertion, but slowly and surely it got easier. The reactions became less severe and I felt less faint. I started to enjoy seeing the world the right way up.

My physio terrorist seemed confident that standing up on my birthday was a possibility, but I knew all too well that nothing was certain when it came to the dreaded Monster.

CHAPTER TWENTY-SEVEN

Breathe Deep, Breathe Deeper

My breathing was feeling like it was more laboured. It started off from when I sat up and I assumed that it was to do with my asthma. But even with an increase in my inhalers, the breathlessness didn't go away, and it started to affect me throughout the day. In fact, it worsened, and I started to get a sharp pain when I inhaled. Within forty-eight hours, it had spread to when I exhaled too. Mum was concerned, so she checked my pulse and temperature.

"Are you nervous, honey?"

"Not really. I just have a pain in my chest."

She looked puzzled and began to hold my wrist again to feel my pulse. Dad entered my room.

"I can feel an ectopic beat. Can you feel this, Col?" Mum said to Dad who held my wrist.

"I can feel an irregular beat," Dad said.

The pain increased over the next few hours, and I felt short of breath. The doctor was called, and as soon as she saw me she was convinced that something was seriously wrong. Although going to hospital was an enormous upheaval, she decided that I needed to be seen by a consultant in A&E.

Dad called for an ambulance, as the pain became acute. Worryingly, they couldn't work out what the pain was either. I tried to explain what it felt like, and I could almost see the alarm bells ringing in their heads. Dad stayed with me until the doctor came, whilst Becky and Mum returned home. All they could think about was what happened to my Gran. She had suffered similar pain but didn't say anything, except for the day before she collapsed, which was too late.

The doctor finally came in the early hours of the morning. She wasn't sure what they were dealing with, but wanted me to be admitted overnight for more investigation. Dad asked the nursing sister where I would be in the morning, as he prepared to go home.

"Oh yes, she's the one with the suspected PE?" the nurse said.

"Pulmonary Embolism? A clot on the lung? No, that's not what we've been told," Dad said.

"Oh, sorry, we'll get back to you," the nurse said as someone called him to another patient.

Dad came back to my bed to say goodbye. "That was confusing. I think they mixed you up with someone else. I'll see you tomorrow, honey."

Once he left, the nurse came into give me some pain relief through my cannula. "The doctor is just coming to see you, Jessica. Don't go to sleep yet."

Within a few minutes, the doctor returned. She stood over my bed and started to talk about the sudden treatment that they needed to do. I desperately tried to understand what she was saying, through my exhaustion.

"I think that you have a Pulmonary Embolism. We have

to give you a big injection of medication to thin your blood so we can disperse it effectively."

A cold sweat filled me. I knew exactly what it was. My Grandma and Grampy had suffered with multiple clots, from Deep Vein Thrombosis to Pulmonary Embolisms.

"We're going to deal with it now and everything should be fine," the doctor said. "Any questions?"

I didn't utter a word, as the stunned silence enveloped me. As she left the cubicle, I was left on my own with just my thoughts to keep me company.

I started texting my family. Cardio problems scared me because my Gran had died from heart problems and my Grandma had died of a blood clotting problem. Why had they waited for Dad to go home before telling me? The bay was silent at 2am in the morning and the darkness was stifling.

Dad replied immediately.

DAD: *Baby, I'm so sorry I wasn't there with you. This is exactly what I didn't want to happen. They'll fix you. Stay calm and Mum will be in with Becky in the morning. Love you more than you could ever know.*

The nurse entered with a big injection to put into my stomach. I had been on smaller doses of the same medication for years, due to my family history. I couldn't sleep. Morbid thoughts kept flicking through my mind. I was texting anyone who was awake, so I wasn't alone. Blissy came online in the early hours of the morning. She had heard from Becky what had happened and she couldn't sleep for fear. Through our messages, I knew that I wasn't on my own—she understood.

BLISSY: *I said to Becky that I would keep talking to you so she could get to sleep for a few hours, then we can swap.*

Despite the fact that I knew Blissy was too poorly to be up all night, she wouldn't leave me. It was a month to go until the date I had planned to stand up, and I knew there was no chance of that happening now. Despite knowing that I was in the best possible hands, I was scared.

It was protocol to be moved on to a ward once you'd been admitted on the Medical Assessment Unit, so I was moved on to the only ward with a spare bed. It was a stroke ward. The bay was filled with ladies who stared at me but couldn't communicate. They were all suffering from Locked-in Syndrome. It was a haunting reminder of what I must have looked like all those years ago.

After a couple of alarming days with specialist tests being done, the doctors confirmed that the massive injection had dispersed the clot. Relief filled me from head to toe. Despite the odd ectopic beat, the pain had gone, I was ready to go home.

Once I got the discharge letter, Mum gave it a quick read. It was filled with medical jargon. The only part that was clear was the need for a follow-up with a consultant who specialised in geriatric care. Mum and I both collapsed into giggles.

"Well honey, at least they are getting you seen by someone with expertise in ageing!"

Although I was only in my twenties, I had to see a doctor who specialised in elderly people. Maybe they were treating me for my bone age, instead of my actual age?

Even though it was a short stay, the hospital admission had exhausted me. I had lived on adrenaline 24/7 and the crash had been inevitable. The stimulation from the hospital had removed all my precious energy that I had been using to get ready to attempt The Long Way Up. It was clear that my goal wasn't going to happen quite as I had planned. Once again, my legs felt like jelly and I was struggling to move my body.

The sound and light that I had endured in the hospital would cause me to suffer with sensory overload for months after I had been discharged. Although it was mentally challenging building up to something that was now not going ahead, it was important for me to know when I had to stop and listen to my body. It would happen another time when I was well enough to manage it.

Tom came to visit a few weeks later, and I wanted to show him that I could sit on the edge of the bed with my legs touching the ground. I always had to choose if I wanted to have a conversation with him or show him my physical improvement—I couldn't do both.

As he sat on my bed, I managed to get up and sit next to him. His eyes widened as he did a double take. It was overwhelming to sit by his side for thirty seconds. He stared at the sister he'd only seen lying down since 2006, and a broad grin appeared on his face.

CHAPTER TWENTY-EIGHT

Long Way Up

In the lead up to the house extension, I contacted Bluewater about doing my sponsored bed push. They gave me a date for fifteen weeks' time and before I knew it, the local news station had asked to cover it in the paper and on TV.

The day before the building was due to commence, I was transferred to Narnia for sixteen weeks of rehabilitation. My hope was that I would have a chance to implement the Long Way Up whilst I was there, with the specialist support from the entire team.

Arriving at Narnia felt like I was coming home; I knew I was completely safe in their care. Dr Nice came in with the physio terrorist, Lucy, who had been assigned to me, to make a plan for what would happen during the stay.

There was a hydrotherapy pool at Narnia and the team decided that it would be my secret weapon in preparing my body to stand up. It was a lot safer for my body to weight bear when I was supported by water.

The first session was planned like a military operation, every part of my journey was considered before I even got into the pool. I was hoisted on to the hydro trolley that would lower me into the water, and a blanket was placed over my head to minimise the effect of the motion. No one would talk to me until I was in the pool, to avoid me using up too much precious energy. As I was lowered down by hydrotherapy assistants, I was submerged in the warm water and I let out a sigh of relief, as my pain significantly eased.

The feeling of the water enabled me to move every part of my body with little effort. The different floats supported my head, as the physio terrorist mobilised the whole of my body. I was able to do so much more in the pool. I even sat up in the water and felt the water act as the support for my frame. After ten minutes of bliss, an exhaustion came over me that made my eyes struggle to stay focused. Within seconds, the team had whipped me out of the pool and transferred me back to my room with a speed that would challenge Usain Bolt.

Over the next few weeks, my physio terrorist and I focused solely on my plan to stand up. Dr Nice tinkered with my medication, to make sure the additional pain I felt from moving more was kept relatively in control.

I felt oddly calm about the stand. I was confident that it would happen but the physio terrorist, Lucy, was more worried about it than I was. First, we had to work out the logistics. I needed to be able to push through my legs and hold my weight. I couldn't even remember how to stand up, or how to connect all the parts of my body to work together to hold my weight, without my bones crumbling from my osteoporosis. Lucy had worked out an action plan that took into consideration every eventuality.

The payback from my hydrotherapy sessions was unforgiving, but I felt elated in all that I achieved in the water. The pain surged through my body and a wave of exhaustion filled every cell of my body. I couldn't have been any more prepared.

The day arrived. Three physio terrorists came to my room. I wore a stabilising belt to take some of the weight and Lucy reminded us all of the plan. Dr Nice was ready to act if necessary, alongside the nurses in case there needed to be a medical intervention. The problem was the unknown—no one knew how my body was going to react. There could be seizures, my bones might not be able to support my own weight. We had to be aware of every situation.

"Are you all ready?" Lucy asked.

A carer started to film and capture every part of this monumental moment. I was as ready as I could ever be. With that, I started step one and sat on the side of the bed. The team watched with anticipation as I took a deep breath and shut my eyes to imagine myself standing up, feeling the weight through my feet, and my quadriceps turning on. Metaphorically, I could hear the cells in my legs heaving my body up. Then I felt my glutes turning on to pull me up with everything I had. What seemed like a long time psyching myself up was a nanosecond in reality.

Lucy pulled on the stability belt and the other physio terrorists assisted my body, the nurses were ready to catch me, and tears of happiness filled Dr Nice's eyes.

I stood up. Just like that. I actually stood up!

A grin filled my face, as I saw the world from a significantly different height. My body supported me. My legs could hold my weight! The whole team started cheering and whooping. A few seconds passed, and my legs turned to jelly, my head started to spin, and the team guided me back to the bed.

The overwhelming joy that filled me was incomparable to anything I had felt before. I had done it! Doctors had said that standing up would never be a possibility. I watched the video on repeat. The magnitude of what I had achieved hit me, the adrenaline ceased, and the exhaustion overcame me.

CHAPTER TWENTY-NINE

For The First Time

The success of a Long Way Up gave me a new-found confidence and hope for the future, despite the horrendous post exertional malaise that I was suffering from.

As soon as Blissy had found out what I had managed, she sent me a special glass engraved with 'The Long Way Up - Mission accomplished.' It made me smile every time I looked at it. It was a constant reminder to never give up. It made me wonder what else was possible. In the past, I had been told that my dream of standing up wouldn't happen but look at me now! Was my body starting to wake up? Or was it getting used to working with a broken battery?

I've spent years being looked after by a multidisciplinary team with a holistic approach to looking after me. The sessions had felt mundane, as if we weren't getting anywhere. Now I realised that every session had been like I was planting a seed, there needed to be the right balance of sun and rain for the seeds to flourish. Seeds grow in all different shapes and sizes. There's often no rhyme or reason to why some do better than others, but the growth will happen in its own time.

The seeds represented my progress. I had planted hundreds

of them since I've been unwell and despite there not always being the right weather to grow, the seeds kept persevering.

My family visited at the weekend and the idea of being able to stand up next to them after all this time, made me feel giddy with excitement. The last time I stood with Becky, she was ten. She was now eighteen years old.

"Becky, come and see this!"

She held my hands and looked at me in disbelief, as she watched me sit up on the edge of the bed, effortlessly. A grin filled her face, as she helped me to get to my feet. It was thirty seconds of pure jubilation as I stood next to her. The emotion flooded over both of us, as we had dreamt of this moment for so long. I gave her a proper hug. My Becky. She was much taller than the last time I stood next to her. She was a young woman now, rather than the scrawny child I remembered.

Suddenly, I was filled with an overwhelming sense of loss, for the time that had passed by in a blink of an eye. I had been so preoccupied with surviving each day with M.E. that I hadn't realised quite how much I had missed out on.

"Thank you for not giving up on me, Becky. I told you that I would do it."

She eased my body back down on to the bed and we both cried. I knew I would remember this moment for the rest of my life.

When I was moved on to the special hydro trolley to go to hydrotherapy, I wondered whether I could use it to transport me to other parts of the hospital. The hydrotherapy was helping me to gain strength in my core, so Lucy had given me the green light to try and increase how long I could sit in a chair, with the hope of venturing outside my one room.

The only problem was that I needed to be reclined a lot to stop my blood pressure from dropping. The wheelchair services had declined me the opportunity to have a specialist wheelchair because, in their eyes, it wouldn't be used enough. But the hydro trolley, which enabled me to lie at a lower incline than if I was in a chair, could be the temporary answer whilst I was at Narnia.

The sponsored bed push was fast approaching, and I needed to try and prepare myself. I hadn't told the team yet, because I knew they would question whether it was something that would cause more harm than good for my body. . . they had a point. I had heightened light and noise sensitivities and I still had to wear industrial strength earplugs every day to survive in my quiet one room. How on earth would I survive the noise of a shopping centre?

It was essential that just like the chair sit and the stand, I broke the task up into manageable bites. The first thing I had to be able to do was to go on short journeys in the hydro trolley, to mimic the ambulance stretcher I would be in.

On the way to one of my appointments, I peered through a gap in the blanket that was covering my head and looked out of the window as we passed. The sun was shining brightly and the sky was bright blue. I had an urge to see what it was like to feel the sun on my face and witness the views outside. I had spent most of the past decade simply dreaming of the outdoors, the fields, trees and flowers. The porter stopped by the door, as he watched my look of wonder. I took a chance and asked him to take me outside.

The sun blinded my eyes from the balcony, as I breathed in the fresh air and looked out at what laid before me. It was the first time I had seen flowers, green grass and trees, since I had become unwell eight years ago. The view went on for as far as my eye could see and I was mesmerised by it. The carers passed the window and took a double take, as they saw me outside of my usual four walls.

As I laid there and enjoyed the view, I decided that I should share the firsts on social media. If I could have shown my fourteen-year-old self the picture of what I was staring at, it would've given me so much hope for the future. A song started playing on my phone called *For the First Time*.

That's it! I thought, I could call it #ForTheFirstTime, and it would start today with a picture of me basking in the sun.

The quick visit outside inspired me to push forwards with attempting to leave my room more often. It gave me such a boost mentally that I knew I needed to keep going, despite how exhausting I found it. The online community was so supportive when I shared the pictures. I wanted to go out in the trolley for a short time once a week—hopefully my energy would be up. Knowing that I wouldn't have to wait long before I could see another view helped me to cope with living within four walls.

My vision for #ForTheFirstTime was to see how many small tasks I could focus on doing that I had once taken for granted. They were simple things like being able to manage my own personal hygiene. For years, I had relied on a carer to wash my face because my arms were too stiff and didn't have the strength to manage it.

I sat up and held the cloth to my face. It was overwhelming to feel my skin for the first time in eight years. I put the cloth into the bowl and then soaked myself. The water filled my pores, which was such an alien sensation to me.

I kept practising for the bed push by going on little rides around the hospital in the hydrotherapy trolley. I was doggedly determined to be able to do it and return to Bluewater. To help with the light sensitivity, I got the carers to open the curtain a bit more for short periods. My eyesight had become quite poor, as it hadn't been stimulated by the light for so long. I turned the television up a little bit louder to get used to more voices. It was all a process and after all this time, I finally felt like I had reached a turning point.

The online community were following the #ForTheFirst-Time moments with elation. In forty-eight hours, they managed to come together to fundraise to buy me my very own recliner wheelchair. The overwhelming kindness of strangers donating to the crowdfunding was immense. To know that people cared so much made all the difference.

On a day I had planned to use the trolley, my physio terrorist Lucy asked me if I would like to try going into one of Narnia's specialist wheelchairs. I was hoisted into the chair and wheeled just outside my room. I hadn't moved in a chair since I was fourteen. All the different stimulations took away my brain power. Although I managed to sit out for ten minutes, my adrenaline left me, causing me to crash hard. My body started to twitch uncontrollably, as it went into paralysis. If determination alone could get M.E. sufferers better, we would all be fully recovered. I needed to remain patient and slow down the pace.

Over the next few weeks, I managed to sit in the chair and reach the bathroom that was just down the corridor. I wanted to increase my tolerance, so I could be transferred into the specialist bath. The bath at Narnia reminded me of the humongous ones that were described in the *Harry Potter* books. I was sure that if I could, I would be able to swim from one end to the other.

The carers hoisted me into the wheelchair and whizzed me into the bathroom, where I was hoisted into the bath. The warm bubbly water soaked my skin. It helped ease the aches and pains, which were blighting my body. I felt instantly relaxed and was reminded of the last time I had a bath, in 2006. I remembered how I had been falling down the stairway of health, and the only thing that I could manage to do was to crawl to the bathroom.

Embarrassingly, Mum and Tom used to help lift me into the bath. I thought of all the time that had passed and the position I was in now. Before I could think about it for any longer, the carers had taken me out of the bath, as my blood pressure had dropped significantly.

In a sense, the Bluewater bed push was my version of climbing Kilimanjaro. It had been a logistical nightmare to plan to go at a time when there would be minimal sensory overload. I was going to do one lap around the huge shopping centre at an off-peak time, with my dad and brother pushing me on an ambulance trolley. Even though I was terrified of how my body would react, I was determined to give it my best shot.

CHAPTER THIRTY

Shop 'Til We Drop

With the bed push only a matter of weeks away, I decided it was time to tell Narnia about it. Many of the carers gasped, whilst other members of the team just shook their heads in disbelief. When I told Dr Nice, he laughed.

"Girls will be girls and girls need to have retail therapy. It's in your DNA. Let's call your trip out a day release! And as usual, we'll be here afterwards for you to rest and recuperate."

On my family's last visit before I went to Bluewater, I decided to surprise them by suggesting that we had lunch out. I got them to push the trolley out into the grounds of Narnia to have a picnic. It felt out of this world to be with them because we hadn't eaten together in over eight years!

Tom and Dad were on their way to take me via ambulance to Bluewater. It felt surreal, as it was the first time I had been in the ambulance with Tom and Dad working as crew mates. Tom had just finished his university degree and was now a qualified paramedic.

"I'll be overtaking the old man soon. Oh, by the way, Stewie is working today otherwise he would've got you to take him out for a drink in Bluewater," Tom said. "You saved yourself a fiver there!"

"I would have only gone for a McDonald's to be fair, so maybe saving a couple of quid," I joked.

"A drink is a drink, mate."

"When are you two going to hook me up with someone? You've both been promising to hitch me up with a man for years."

"Mate, we are trying but. . ." Tom looked away.

"Nobody would want someone who has my kind of problems." I sighed.

"No, you're my sister and you've been through enough shit with that arsehole who abused you in that hospital."

Jackson had been a carer who took advantage of me when I was sixteen years old. As much as I had struggled to come to terms with everything that happened, my family had too. Mum and Dad had thought I was safe in that hospital, but then their worst nightmare came true.

"I'm not letting someone take advantage of you again, mate. Big bro rules there." Tom smiled.

As the ambulance started the journey to Bluewater, every effort was made to try and create as little stimulation as possible. I wore a blanket over my head, whilst I breathed in the Entonox, I needed all the energy I could muster to survive the sensory overload that was coming my way. It was going to be an important moment for me. A local news team wanted to do a video of the bed push, as it seemed extraordinary that I hadn't been shopping in so long.

I was brought into Bluewater Shopping Centre through the staff entrance. As Tom and Dad pushed the trolley through the maze of corridors, butterflies filled my stomach. We came out to the front of John Lewis and to my surprise, there was a crowd huddled together. When they saw me, they started to whoop and cheer.

For a moment, I thought I recognised some of them. I hadn't told anyone the time we were going to get there but all my local family and friends had come to support me and keep my morale high. I hadn't seen most of these people since before I had become unwell, but it was as if I had seen them only yesterday.

The glass ceiling was painfully bright, as it reflected the sky. Even though they weren't the most charming accessory, I kept the ear defenders on tightly, as Tom and Dad pushed the ambulance trolley slowly around the shopping centre. When I passed certain shops, I was reminded of the memories I had of being at Bluewater, particularly the times I had been with Gran. I briefly looked up and the sky was a clear blue. Her favourite colour. I was sure she was looking down on me with a smile.

The staff made sure I had come at the quietest moment. It was a Sunday, so the shops opened later and were relatively empty. The only sound was that of my supporters cheering me onwards. It was cognitively exhausting to adjust to all the lights and sound, it took all my strength to keep going. We managed to go into a shop with the trolley, and I bought a bottle of orange juice. To actually give the cashier the money and leave the shop with a bag felt immense.

Five minutes later my body began to crash terribly, as the M.E. Monster snarled at me for having some enjoyment. I was no longer coherent and I started to lose the ability to move. I had gone from being enthralled to share this moment with so many people, to a shadow of myself in searing agony. Tom and Dad quickly steered the trolley away from everyone, just as I began to fade into Limbo Land. The images of my concerned friends filled my mind and I could hear their hushed voices.

"Oh god! She's really not well."

"Bless her, she looks really underweight. Poor love."

I laid in the back of the ambulance, as Dad opened the bottle of orange juice to give me a couple of sips.

"You did it, kiddo. Remember that moment every time you need to be reminded of how far you've come," Dad said.

When I returned to Narnia, I rested as much as I could. I dozed in and out of conscious thought, existing through every minute and hour. Ordinarily, these moments of payback would've lasted weeks and months, but this time it was for much less. Adrenaline still swamped me whenever I thought of the mammoth task I had just completed. I couldn't believe that so much had changed in one year.

I felt a buzz knowing that not only had it been a massive achievement for me, but I had also raised a lot of sponsorship money for Share a Star. This came at the same time as Share a Star became a fully registered charity. I couldn't believe that the little idea formed in 2010 had grown and flourished into something so special.

Everyone at Narnia marvelled at what I had managed. They had seen me at my most vulnerable, when I hadn't been able to cope with the light from a slight gap in the curtain, and couldn't listen to music, let alone a crowd talking.

I was starting to prepare to return home. It was daunting but exciting to be coming back to so much change. I ended the last day at Narnia on a high when I proudly managed to brush my teeth on my own whilst sitting up.

My little project #ForTheFirstTime had not only raised awareness for severe M.E., but it had made people appreciate what they had in a way they hadn't thought of before. I was rejoicing in being able to do something they didn't have to even think about, like going to the bathroom to brush their teeth and wash their face. I didn't want anyone else to have to lose everything like I had.

I waved goodbye to all the staff at Narnia, as Dad and Kip pushed the trolley to the ambulance. Dad spent the journey describing to me my new room downstairs and what the kitchen now looked like.

When we got home, instead of the horrendous heave to get me upstairs, I could be wheeled up the path and straight into my new room. I took a moment to take in the newly painted walls and all the furniture that I had chosen. My world of one room had been upgraded and now looked amazing. This room was going to be the start of new adventures.

CHAPTER THIRTY-ONE

Spread The Hope

Being back home with Team Taylor was wonderful, but getting used to being downstairs in the centre of the family house was challenging. Unlike upstairs, noise came from all directions. There was the washing machine, the tumble dryer, people banging kitchen appliances around and everyone having multiple conversations. It was hard to rest, as every noise made me jump and pierced my ears.

Despite the ongoing torture that the M.E. Monster caused, I had been planning for an exciting new musical opportunity. Music was such a big part of my life before I was ill. It had been my passion. I used to enjoy singing harmonies in the church choir and coming up with new songs from a young age. I played the violin and the clarinet, but I had always loved the piano. I used to listen to Tom playing in the living room and when he left the music sheets, I tried to teach them to myself.

When I was in hospital in 2010, I came up with an idea for a Christmas song. I had barely been able to tolerate the sound of any music, so I used to imagine it playing in my head. Christmas had always been my favourite time of the year and I loved that the music was timeless.

The melody went around my head, whilst I came up with some lyrics to go with it. I called it *Spread the Hope*, and over many months I recorded it on my phone. When I sent it to Mum, she shared with our musical friends who said they wanted to make it come alive.

Many years after I had help to arrange the song, my old violin teacher volunteered his daughter and one of my oldest friends, Elizabeth, to do the vocals. She recorded it whilst I was at Narnia and wanted to come and show it to me. It was going to be the first time I had seen her since I had been struck down with the M.E. Monster. I hadn't really seen any of my friends due to how unpredictable my health was. I had tried to make plans to meet up with Elizabeth, but the Monster had always intervened and prevented it from happening.

When she arrived, she looked completely different to how I had remembered her eight years ago. I hadn't seen my violin teacher in even longer and for a moment, we didn't know what to say to each other. So much had happened since I had last seen them; I was a different girl to the one they remembered. It was as if I had been through a war zone. I found it hard to be as quick-witted as I used to be. The reality was we had all grown up.

We hugged each other closely, not wanting to let go. The last time we'd seen each other was when we were teenagers going through a dodgy 'emo stage,' with black hair and very pale skin.

I had known Elizabeth since I was born. We used to sing together and went to the same Primary School. It was hard to see her and know that I wasn't able to do all of things we used to do together. I hadn't finished school and gone to wild parties with her. It was a new level of grief for the life that had been taken from me, and what I wished I was able to do.

It was still exciting to put our plans into action. I couldn't sing anymore due to the sheer energy it took but Elizabeth was the perfect person for the job. She was used to performing and her voice was beautiful, much better than mine had ever been. They sat down and played me the recording of *Spread the Hope*.

The haunting mix of Elizabeth's voice with the piano and cello filled my heart. It was even better than I imagined it would be. Even though it was August, I was already excited to hear it at Christmas time.

After meeting up with Elizabeth, I promised myself that I would keep meeting with my friends, despite the energy that it took. I had gone without seeing the friends that I loved for years, due to the advice given by one of the hospitals I was in. They said it would make me worse, and that I needed to focus my energy on getting better. But even though I followed what they said, I hadn't become drastically better. In some ways, I just became more isolated and lonelier over the years.

I've spent so long simply existing in the same four walls but having someone different enter every so often made me feel like I was living. It meant the M.E. Monster wasn't controlling my entire life.

Since returning home from Narnia, I tried to maintain my improvement by standing up when I had the energy to do so. As there weren't as many health professionals at home, Dad and my carer would put a stabilising belt around me and a Zimmer frame to assist me. There was nothing like being in my twenties and having to be hunched over like an old lady to steady myself!

I listened to *Spread the Hope* regularly and hearing it come to life continued to inspire me. Listening to music was a different sound to that of the everyday noises that hurt my ears. Music made me feel alive and when I listened to the piano, I could almost imagine my fingers playing along.

I felt a hunger to be able to escape my one room. Now that I was downstairs, this felt like a tangible goal. Whilst I was still waiting for my new recliner wheelchair to be delivered, I asked to be hoisted into a reclining shower chair, so I could see what the ground floor of my house looked like since the extension work had been done.

My carer pushed the seat out into the kitchen and to the front room. I hadn't seen the living room in eight long years. It had been the place where we had all sat as a family to watch the television. We'd lived in this house since I was three years old.

The room hadn't changed. The white walls and the settees were the same as when I had left. The last time I had been in the living room was when I had started to become unwell. I would lie down on the sofa with a duvet wrapped around me. As the weeks passed, the room became darker and darker, as my light sensitivity grew. The day I had been forced to stop going to school by the wretched M.E. Monster, I had laid in this room cuddled up to Becky.

It wasn't just about seeing another room, it showed me that I was on my way back, and I was making progress in big ways. I was starting to make headway in getting my life back from the M.E. Monster after years of continuous suffering.

The arrival of my brand-spanking-new wheelchair was a

game changer. I had a list of things I wanted to try and do to continue my #ForTheFirstTime project. I couldn't wait to be hoisted into it to try it out.

The first place I wanted to go was the garden. My carer pushed me into the new kitchen and through the back door. The fresh air was crisp and sharp. All the memories of the last time that I was in the garden played out in my mind. Becky's laughter as we played in the long summer evenings. Now the Wendy house and trampoline that Becky had played with was gone, highlighting how much she had continued to grow up without me.

I sat there for five whole minutes before my energy was zapped from me. When I first got ill, I was embarrassed to use a wheelchair, now it felt miraculous. Once I got back to my room, I warmly embraced Dad.

"It was amazing! It was just incredible. I saw outside."

The payback was immediate and I had to be hoisted back to my bed before I collapsed.

I had to build up my strength to use the wheelchair to visit the living room again. I looked at the piano sitting in the corner. It hadn't been played since I had been ill and I had a sudden urge to go over to it. I desperately wanted to feel the black and white keys underneath my fingers, even though it was difficult to get close to it in my chair.

My carer held on my hand and guided it to the notes. When I reached out and touched a key, it made such a satisfying sound. To my surprise, it didn't hurt when I pushed down on the key, in fact, it made me feel warm inside.

My hands reached to the keys that I had last played in 2006, and my subconscious took over. I began to play the beginning of *The Glasgow Love Theme* from *Love Actually*. Becky and Mum stood silently listening to me, as they took in the moment we'd all been waiting for. I played for around thirty seconds, until exhaustion fogged over me. I was hoisted back into the bed just before I crashed following the effort it had taken to play.

Managing to play the piano had opened my eyes to what else I could do now I had a suitable wheelchair. I wanted to decorate the Christmas tree with a bauble. When we were younger, we'd always decorated the tree as a family. Arguing over what the colour coordination would be symbolised the start of the festive season in our family. Christmas hadn't been the same since we'd spent most of them in hospital, let alone after Gran's fatal heart attack seven years ago. This year was going to be one to remember.

It was the evening of the Upnor Carol Service when we decided to put the Christmas tree up. Becky was taken aback that I was able to help, after so many years of doing it alone. Being able to get into another room was not something I took for granted anymore.

As I glimpsed at the tree and decorations, I wanted to savour every moment of this year's festive season. Becky switched the Christmas songs on to quietly play *Spread the Hope*. She wheeled me towards the tree that stood in the middle of the room, with white lights twinkling around it. I chose a star from the box of baubles on the sofa and she guided my hand to hang it on a branch.

"Spread the Hope throughout the world, bring the light into somebody's life, give the message this Christmas time, that it's gonna be alright."

Elizabeth's voice filled my mind as I reflected on my year. I started the year in hospital. I had been stuck in a world of one room upstairs, with no chance of being able to find my freedom. Now, I had just put a bauble on the Christmas tree, listening to my own song playing on the audio system! If that wasn't showing the M.E. Monster who was boss, then I don't know what could.

There was a card from Tom and Jem waiting for me to open. As I opened it, the paper-cut snowflake fell out of the envelope. The words read 'Will you be my bridesmaid?'

I screamed, "Yes!"

Becky came into the room holding her snowflake. Tom had stuck to his end of the bargain by giving me time to get better and it was my turn to think of a plan to attend his wedding.

2015

CHAPTER THIRTY-TWO

Smile For A Smile

The payback from the festivities made me feel like I had succumbed to the Monster of my nightmares. I had tried to sit in my chair because I desperately didn't want my autonomic system to crash again, but I had to stop because it felt like I was drowning in exhaustion. I was too fatigued to even understand what my carer was saying. It was as if she were speaking a foreign language at a hundred miles per hour. When I tried to answer her, my mind went blank and no words came out. It was beyond frustrating.

Then there were the absent moments that were becoming more frequent. If I over-exerted, my hands would shake as I tried to move them. My mind would go completely blank as if the Monster were taking control of my whole body. That was what made this illness so terrifying—I could deteriorate so quickly and without much warning.

My social media family were incredible. They sent supportive messages to me when I was quiet and they surprised me with gifts to keep my spirits up. I really was so lucky to have them. Blissy sent me a postcard with the word SMILE written in capital letters. Even though I was suffering considerably more,

I chose to smile. The card reminded me that I could smile in defiance to show the M.E. Monster that although it could do many things, it couldn't take away my hope.

I woke up feeling intensely unwell. I couldn't concentrate or function cognitively. My carer came into my room to give me a drink. I tried to focus on her but the pungent smell of her perfume made me feel sick. The sound of her voice made me wince as it echoed around my head. I felt like I was crashing, the world was becoming more and more distant, and my mind was empty. It could have been Limbo Land, but it felt even further away than that. It was like. . . I had gone.

Voices reverberated around me, but I couldn't tell who they were.

"She's fitting! Help me! She has gone completely stiff!" A female voice shouted.

"Oh my God! Get her on her side. Darling Jessica, hold on."
Where was I?

My mind was numb. I couldn't think. I couldn't breathe.
Where was I?

"Tom, it's not stopping. It's not stopping. Why won't it stop?" A shrill female voice cried.

"Call an ambulance. She needs to go into hospital. Quickly! Call 999."

Who was that? Where the hell am I? Questions whirled around my empty brain. *I'm so tired. . . so very, very tired.*

"Ambulance, it's my daughter. She's been in a seizure for too long," the female voice said urgently. "She looks grey and her lips are going blue."

"The shaking. . . the shaking. . . I mean yes, but she's struggling to because she is shaking so vigorously."

I'm in pain. . . so much pain. . . everywhere. . . everywhere.

There were more voices and more noise pulsating around me.

"How long has this been going on for?" a male voice asked.

"Nearly twenty minutes. We rolled her on her side, but I don't know what else to do."

"Pulse 130. Temperature 37. Oxygen level's a bit low," another male voice said.

"Jessica, I'm one of the paramedics. We're just going to put this mask on to help you breathe. We need to give you some medication. One's called diazepam and needs to go up into your bottom. We're going to make you better."

Who are they? Where am I? The voices became fainter.

"Change of plan, mate. Let's just get her into hospital. We aren't going to manage to stop it and we are wasting precious time," someone said. "Okay, Jessica, we're going to move you on to the stretcher and take you to A&E. We need to get you better."

Noises. Sirens. More voices. . . more people. So loud. . . it hurts. . . so tired. . . so much pain. . . so. . . very. . . tired.

"We need to keep her airway open. Put a tube in," a voice said.

"Turn the oxygen up high," another said. "Give her some stronger anti-convulsion drugs."

"I think we need to use phenytoin," a female voice stated.

"Shit. I bloody *hate* that drug. Do you remember what happened to the last patient I had to give it to?" a male voice groaned.

"Give it to her quickly. If that doesn't stop the seizure, we will have to intubate,"

I tried to speak but groans were all that left me.

My head. . . where am I? Mum? Becky? Dad? The pain. . . the pain in my body. . . So exhausted. . . just so tired. . . too tired. . . too heavy. . . sounds and noises. . . Mum? Becky? Dad? Where am I? Tell me where I am!

My body felt like a tonne of bricks as I tried to move my limbs. All I could hear was the sound of voices talking urgently to one another.

"Up her dose of the phenytoin," the same female voice said.

"Only if you're sure," a male voice sighed.

As I tried to open my eyes, bright white lights filled my blurred vision. The noise from the machines filled my ears. I must be in hospital. I was too exhausted to think. The M.E. Monster snarled and began to protest at the lights and noise that surrounded me.

Once I started to focus and twitch at different noises, the male voice spoke quietly to me. "Jessica, I want you to keep breathing slowly. The oxygen mask will help you do that. I need you to keep calm. You're in hospital because you had a prolonged seizure. I'm the nurse who's been looking after you. You've been given a lot of strong medication that will make you feel rough, so we need you to rest."

I nodded, my head was spinning and I fell into a dazed rest. A hand was stroking my forehead and I could hear the deep voice of my dad. He hugged me. I could faintly see Becky stood on the other side of the bed. The relief filled their faces, as I managed to smile at them.

"Yes, Jessica! That smile brightens up the room. We all needed to see that," Dad said before I closed my eyes and fell into a deep sleep.

CHAPTER THIRTY-THREE

Send A Smile

I was discharged from the ward a few days later. The NHS had been exemplary. Becky told me about how the paramedics, alongside the resuscitation team, had saved my life. It made me feel truly humbled to still be here, surviving every minute that passed. The neurologists thought that I had secondary epilepsy due to the severity of my M.E. and with a list of new medications, I was allowed to return home.

Kip and Dad picked me up from hospital. Dad sat in the back of the ambulance with me and connected me to the Entonox. My body felt like it had run a double marathon and my limbs felt like lead.

I deteriorated just a week later and the familiar unwell feeling washed over me again. The colour drained from my face and I was drenched in a cold sweat. I heard more voices being called, as I slipped in and out of consciousness. My body was taking me to a new level of crashing. I desperately tried to call out, but a load of mumbled nonsense words were all that left my mouth. Then I was gone: Limbo Land engulfed me.

My body felt like it had been hit by a bus. I let my brain

float through my thoughts because I was too exhausted to keep swimming; I needed to just survive. My body was temporarily broken but seeing my family and holding them close instilled a calmness in me. I felt so far away from where I had been just six months ago.

The doctor came to my house and said that getting the balance of medication right to prevent the seizures from happening again was a bit of an experiment. Meanwhile, I was encouraged to rest.

The more I laid there in my one room, the more isolated I felt. The prolonged seizure had left me feeling like I was on an emotional rollercoaster. When I tried to sleep, my dreams took me back to resus and the urgent voices of the medics haunted me.

"We've tried everything."

"She's been in this seizure for too long, we have to intubate her."

When I wasn't reliving my worst nightmare I had to try and occupy my mind and think of something I could do. All my online friends had flooded me with get well soon messages. They made such a difference to my life.

I noticed Blissy's postcard on the windowsill and the word 'SMILE' was staring at me. Then the idea came to me. Throughout the past few weeks, people's smiles had helped me so much—Dad's smile when I gained consciousness had calmed me down. Becky's smile was a constant reassurance and even when I had been terrified, people smiling at me made me feel better. It didn't matter where in the world you lived or what language you spoke—a smile was universal.

My idea was to take a picture of me smiling and send it to

someone online, which would then in turn make them smile. If that person then took a picture of themselves smiling and passed it on, the smile would keep on travelling.

So with the help of my family and my carer, I recorded a short video. This was the start of Send a Smile for a Smile. Even though my seizures didn't stop, seeing other people's smiles filling the online community was incredible. People from all over the world got involved and it made me realise that we're all connected to each other.

Stewie came round to see me. "You alright, Butt Munch?" He smiled at me and gave me a hug. "Now I wasn't expecting my colleague and friend to be coming out to you. I know you really want a boyfriend, but there is no need to go to the extent of calling an ambulance to get one!"

I cringed at the thought that one of his friends had had to put medication into an intimate part of my body.

"Why do you know every single paramedic in Medway?" I asked.

"Because I work in the area, so I literally know everyone."

I raised my eyebrows at his taunts and laughed. "Well, if you'd hurry up and find me someone suitable then there would be no problem."

"True, but I have just come up with an ingenious plan, my friend. What about internet dating?"

"Err, no, that won't work," I moaned.

"It will! You're always saying how important the online community is. Now, let's use it."

I looked sceptically at him. "Really? Do we have to?"

"Yes, we do. I'll write your profile. I'll even pay for it because I'm a gent." He downloaded the App on my phone and wrote a suitable profile for me. "If it works for you, then you can sign me up, now that I'm single again."

After he left I spent time looking at different profiles online. I felt strangely self-conscious, as I wondered if this was going to help. *Who would want me?* I didn't actually go outside. I couldn't do things for myself. I lived in a bed for goodness sake! But I could hear Stewie's voice saying that was the right place to be.

There were some interesting men, but one called Samuel Bearman caught my eye. He swiped on my profile and started to talk to me. He seemed nice, but I wondered why he was using internet dating as well. Samuel would talk to me even when I went quiet. He kept messaging me and asking about my M.E. and it didn't seem to faze him that I was ill. This was a good sign. Maybe I had found someone who I could meet up with? But the whole idea made me feel vulnerable.

I sighed, why have Jackson's actions affected my confidence now?

Hopefully, Samuel would make the first move, even if it was just with a smile.

CHAPTER THIRTY-FOUR

WAV

The new medication that the doctors put me on to try and control the seizures made me feel so drugged that my brain felt numb. I couldn't think. I couldn't speak without slurring. The medics were baffled by the convulsions and wanted me to be seen in a specialist hospital. My body was always a medical mystery, but I decided to email Dr Nice at Narnia to ask him for his opinion. He responded back quickly.

Hello Jessica!
Those seizures do sound horrendous. A small percentage of the very severe M.E. cases I have dealt with have had seizures as you describe—maybe not quite as long as yours though. The problem is, if it is due to the M.E. then the treatments won't work and when you have more tests, it probably won't show up.
Wish I had better news for you. Keep hanging in there.
Dr Nice

The multiple blue light ambulance trips to A&E had given me a new understanding with regards to the families that my charity Share a Star helped. The fear and uncertainty of when the next emergency would happen was something they had to deal with on a daily basis.

I wanted to try and be there for those families in their time of need. Share a Star had supported a lot of seriously unwell children in the time it had been running. There was one local boy we'd helped when he was in a life and death situation. Even though my health was a struggle, I had managed to keep in touch with the family. To my surprise, his mum broke down on the radio when she mentioned about how invaluable Share a Star's support had been.

"Jessica was always there. It's hard being in a hospital on your own, spending every minute of every day watching your son connected to machines. I have three other young children at home, and I felt awful not being there, but Share a Star made them smile when I couldn't. There are no words for what Share a Star and Jessica did for me."

What started as a little idea of making seriously unwell children into stars had done far more than I had ever anticipated it would. Then I came up with an idea—*would it be possible to connect with her to work together to help more families?*

My old school contacted me to raise funds to send some severely unwell children and their families on special outings. I felt a mixture of emotions because I hadn't heard from them since I was forced to suddenly leave early in 2006. It was a high-achieving grammar school, and I knew that the pressure all the students were under caused a lot of them to become physically and mentally unwell.

Even though my deterioration in health had been clear, many of my teachers just thought I was being lazy when I had to lie my head down on the desk during lessons. They thought I was being disrespectful, when I actually needed their help. Despite it being a challenging school setting, I made lots of friends when I was there but they were at university now, and once again I was left behind.

My school held a Founder's Day service every year at Rochester Cathedral. All the teachers, present and past students would attend the celebration. There was music from the school orchestra, hymns and a teaching from the Bishop of Rochester. This year, they wanted someone to come and talk to the students about what the school fundraising for Share a Star would be used on.

It had never been an option for me to leave my house. The only time I had left my room in the past nine years was when an emergency ambulance had taken me to hospital. My occupational health therapist and physio terrorist happened to be in the room when my old teacher phoned about the service.

"I'll have to try and find someone to come because, I mean, I haven't left my house for years," I said.

But the therapists looked at each other and then at me. They whispered to each other and I couldn't concentrate on my phone call. I had never been particularly accomplished at multitasking.

"You look as if you've both come up with an idea," I said warily once the call had ended.

"It is an idea, well a plan, a cunning one at that," the occupational health therapist said. "We're working towards you getting to your brother's wedding, aren't we? I think it's time we got you used to a car. You won't be going to the wedding in an ambulance. You're going to have a WAV, which is a wheelchair accessible vehicle, but you need to get used to it. What about if our goal is getting you to the Founder's Day?"

I grinned from ear to ear. "That would be amazing! I didn't even know that was an option."

"Your wheelchair has opened up your world. You're not completely trapped in one room anymore. You can be hoisted into it and I don't think it will be long before you can transfer from bed to chair without the hoist. We're going to build up that strength. A WAV will completely change your life. You could go out and watch the outside world. You can get somewhere if you need to but most importantly we want you to get to Tom's wedding and you need to build up to it. So I think we have got a plan of action," the physio terrorist said.

Mum and Dad started looking at different WAVs that would suit my specific needs. It was essential that I could lie down, that the windows were dark so there was minimal light and it needed to have good suspension too. We had to do a test drive to make sure it was suitable for me to survive an hour and a half drive to the wedding destination in Hampshire.

I was excited to get in the WAV and go on a test drive. It made me feel like I was one step closer to getting to the wedding. Whenever I spoke to Tom and Jem on the phone, they told me of their plans to make the wedding accessible for me. I desperately wanted to get there. I had missed so much since the M.E. Monster had come into my life, but I wasn't prepared to miss this.

Dad showed me pictures of the car they were going to test drive. It was a van with a specialist ramp and a winch that would attach to my wheelchair, so it could pull me into the car.

A big vehicle didn't faze Dad because he was used to driving ambulances around.

Once I was hoisted into my chair, I was wrapped in blankets. The light was too much even with my dark glasses on, so my face was covered with a sheet. The winch was connected to my wheelchair and I was pulled up the ramp into the car. It wasn't a particularly pleasant experience because it felt like my wheelchair was going to go over even though the chair and I were strapped in tightly.

Dad started the car and I could feel the vibrations of the engine tingle in my body. I thought that my ear defenders would be enough, but I hadn't anticipated the extent of the noise. Whenever I had been in an ambulance, I had Entonox to dull my senses. Unfortunately, that was only used in ambulances and hospital settings.

In the car, every bump in the road reverberated around my body. I didn't think it was possible to feel exhausted by feeling motion. I was wrong. I pulled the sheet slightly away from my eye, so I could see through the window. I watched as we passed the old haunts around my family home. When I was in an ambulance, it was impossible to see out of the windows. Seeing the familiar trees and fields made me smile, because it was the first time I had seen them in such a long time.

My joy didn't last because the motion made me feel sick. I felt so exhausted that I couldn't take in what was passing by the window. I began to feel dizzy, so I placed the blanket back over my face. The noise of the vehicle agitated me, as the sensory overload filled my body. It had only been a five-minute journey, but that was enough.

Mum noticed my body was starting to crash and told

Dad to get home quickly. My consciousness started to fade as exhaustion came over me. Even when we arrived home and the car was stationary, I couldn't move or murmur a sound. We sat in silence as Mum checked my pulse and made sure I wasn't having a seizure. The only link we'd found with my seizures is that I tended to have more of them when I was exhausted.

Even though I crashed, we decided the car model was suitable for me. The car was made and adapted as soon as the order came in and it took a long time to sort out. The car would be delivered the same day as the Founder's Day and I couldn't help but think that God was making sure I went to Rochester Cathedral for the service.

CHAPTER THIRTY-FIVE

Founder's Day

I was preparing my speech with Becky, when Mum came bounding into the room holding the phone receiver in her hand.

"Guess who has just rung, Jessica?"

I had no idea and was in the middle of trying to describe my memories from my school days and how they shaped my future. I didn't have time to play games.

"You have been nominated and *shortlisted*. . ."

I looked up wondering how I've been shortlisted for anything.

"For The Pride of Britain Awards for your charity work!"

What? I had never been nominated for anything before and I couldn't contemplate as to why I was being considered worthy for such an accolade.

The Pride of Britain is an annual awards ceremony held to celebrate the unsung heroes in the United Kingdom. How could I possibly be worthy of that?

Whilst I continued to work on my speech, Samuel messaged me on the dating app. I really liked him. He didn't mind when I was unable to be in touch. He was just always there. At first,

I didn't want to explain to him that I was disabled and bed bound ninety-nine percent of the time.

When Stewie had set up the dating app for me, I made sure that my M.E. wasn't mentioned. I didn't want to be judged on that, as I was pretty sure that most men would run a mile with the baggage I came with.

But I felt that I could tell Samuel anything. When I finally plucked up the courage to tell him that I was housebound, he told me that that was fine! He preferred to stay in than go out. I explained that it was due to a chronic illness that had blighted me since I was a teenager and he looked up the disease so he knew more about it. Nothing fazed him and that made me feel even more attracted to him.

Both of us really want to meet in person. We decided that we would make a plan to meet *after* I had done my first speech to two thousand people at Rochester Cathedral as that in itself felt like more than enough to contemplate.

On the morning of the Founder's Day service, I had to be up early. I always felt worse in the mornings, so it was a task for me to wake up. I had butterflies in my stomach as I tried to master my nerves. My new car was due to be delivered in the morning to take me to the cathedral. It arrived just in time for me to be quickly loaded into it and we were off. The adrenaline that I felt all morning due to the terror of delivering a speech to so many people, masked the nausea and sensory overload that I felt with the motion of the ride.

I have to get there, I thought.

On the way, Mum and Becky were discussing what we should call our new car.

"It needs to have a good name," Mum said.

"Then I'm the person for the job! I'm pretty damn good at coming up with names for inanimate objects," Becky said.

"So, what is it going to be then?"

"Well I think it should be an old-fashioned name that we can't forget." Becky grinned. "I hereby announce that this car will be called Brenda Bus!"

When we arrived, we were ushered to our seats on the front row. I felt like everyone was looking at me because I was the only person in a wheelchair. The service started and I was flooded with memories of when I had been a student. It hadn't really changed since I had last attended and a strange nostalgia filled me. We used to sit together in classes and would spend our time purposely changing the words of the school song as we sang it. The teachers would hiss down the row, telling us to behave ourselves but we wouldn't listen.

The second hymn was already halfway through when I came out of my reveries. I mouthed along to the hymn, too embarrassed to try singing with my damaged vocals. Before I knew it, my name was introduced and a sea of two thousand heads stared towards me. The silence was deafening and my heart was hammering in my chest. I made my way to the stage, faced the sea of people, took a deep breath and began to tell my story.

Some teachers came up to congratulate me afterwards. Some hadn't recognised me at all, but I forgave them as it was fair to say that I had physically changed a lot since they had taught me. The young students who had been sitting where I had, nine years previously, had been inspired to raise money to support our cause. I felt protective of them because I wanted them to realise how important their health was. When I had sat there, I had no inkling as to where my life would lead me. I wanted them to grasp every opportunity and live in a way I wished I had the chance to.

Recovering from my trip to Rochester Cathedral was painfully slow. My noise sensitivity had heightened since I listening to the whole school and an orchestra singing hymns. I desperately wanted to meet Samuel. He was so supportive since I started talking to him but my parents were concerned about me meeting up with someone from the internet. No matter how long ago I had suffered the abuse at the hands of Jackson, my parents still worried about me around men.

"You're a vulnerable adult Jessica. You just need to be sure," Mum said when I first told her and Dad about Samuel.

Mum and Dad listened to me talk on the phone to Samuel every evening. We'd talk for hours about absolutely everything. He was so down to earth and we enjoyed the same music and films and had similar core values about the importance of family.

I saved up all my energy so we could talk into the night on Messenger. My parents could see that I was the most content that I had been since becoming unwell.

CHAPTER THIRTY-SIX

The First Date

A few weeks later, Samuel and I arranged for him to come down to Kent from Essex to meet me. I spent the morning getting ready with the help of my carer. She helped me apply my makeup and do my hair. I wanted to look my best, and as I looked into the mirror that my carer was holding, I could feel the butterflies in my stomach multiplying.

I had never met someone new in my one room before, let alone a guy that I had feelings for. I was anxious that my health would let me down. He was going to see my disability before he met me. Would he treat me differently once he realised how disabled I was?

Samuel didn't drive and the nearest train station was a couple of miles away from our house. There was no other choice but to have the awkward situation of Dad picking him up and meeting him before me. I spoke to Dad many times in the week leading up to Samuel coming down. When I thought of all the embarrassing stories that he'd told Becky's first boyfriend, I became paranoid to make sure the same didn't happen to me.

As he went to pick Samuel up, I went over it one more time

before he left; I was desperate for Dad not to scare Samuel off before I had even met him.

"No questions! Don't make any of your normal dad jokes, and he'll probably be really quiet. Promise me you won't scare him away? Dad?"

"Don't worry, I'll wait in the car until he finds me. I'll say hello but I won't ask him any questions about his journey or how much he likes my daughter and I will definitely not scare him by saying anything about what I will do if he hurts you. I think that's everything you've been telling me for the past week?" He laughed and went to leave the room.

"Dad, just be cool, okay?" I pleaded.

"You got it."

Ten minutes later, Dad walked up the garden path, accompanied by a quiet young man who followed sheepishly behind him. As they entered my room, my heart skipped a beat. It was the first time I had been on a date since the M.E. Monster had taken over my life.

He was painfully shy and I could see that he was having to fight against his own anxiety. Other than being a bit shorter than I expected, he looked as I had envisaged. I wondered what his first thoughts were about me?

He was rooted to the spot with nerves and for a brief moment we didn't know what to say to each other. I found his shyness oddly endearing because I knew that getting on a train to meet a stranger must have taken a lot of bravery. He puts his hands on to the bed rail and they were shaking violently.

"Here you go Samuel, here she is. We're just going to go to the cinema, so will leave you to it." Dad patted Samuel on the arm before turning to me. "I've got my phone on me and. . . err. . . Agnes will be in the other room if you need her."

We'd made a decision that we would try to code my carer's name because I was self-conscious about the fact I needed someone with me at all times. I would need to ask for my carer to help with toileting and feeding whilst Samuel was there, and I felt embarrassed to have to ask for constant assistance for my basic needs. I didn't want to overwhelm Samuel with my complex health needs. Today had to be perfect.

Dad left the room and I tried to not look nervous, but I was desperate to make sure that Samuel saw beyond the fact I was stuck in a bed. I was just a girl on a date. He tried to start a conversation, but his nerves took his breath away. *Maybe I wasn't what he expected?*

I suddenly realised that he was looking for somewhere to sit. The room was full of medical equipment and the chair by my bed looked like it had just come out of a hospital. No wonder he looked confused!

"You can sit there. It's just a normal chair, but a tad less comfortable."

He grinned and sat down awkwardly on the chair. He began to chat and show me the list of films that he'd brought for us to watch and food he had managed to find.

"I got you some popcorn because everyone needs popcorn when they watch a film. Plus, I thought that might be easier to eat, and I can always help you." His cheeks went scarlet as I could see him wondering whether he had said the right thing. "I did check that you wouldn't be allergic to it but double check it. I don't want our first date to end up with an allergic reaction."

I laughed. "No I think I have probably weirded you out

enough with this room. I mean the hoist above my head is just the icing on top of the cake, don't you think?"

"No, I would say the icing was having to meet your dad before you and sit in silence on the trip here!"

I groaned as I felt my cheeks getting hot. "Yep, what a welcome to the wonderful world of Jessica. I hate my body!"

"Well, I like it, so there's no need to worry."

A warm feeling filled my insides like I had never felt before, and I smiled at him.

"I'm sure that you weren't really expecting all this when I said I'm often bed bound. Bed with bars on it and surrounded with medical equipment."

"The good thing about bars is that when I'm cuddling up to you watching one of these films, I won't fall out of the bed and embarrass myself! Anyway, the bed wins for comfort too—I always get a stiff back when I'm trying to watch a film at the cinema. Oh, and by the way the medical equipment is a unique accessory."

He came and laid next to me on my bed. We watched the latest *X-Men* film. He cuddled into me and I put my hand on his and leant my head on to his shoulder. It was the happiest I had felt for years.

I needn't have worried about Samuel being scared away by my health issues. He was not fazed by the fact that I asked him to help me sit up and left the room when I needed my carer to help me. The time we had together seemed to fly by and before long, Mum and Dad came back from the cinema.

"We're back! Didn't you say that you needed to get the train at 4:30pm Samuel?" Dad called.

I looked at Samuel and we both sighed.

"Well this sucks but I have to go. Sunday service trains are awful." He kissed me softly on my cheek. My insides began to squirm with happiness. "This has been amazing. The best day and I can't wait to do it again. Maybe we will actually finish the film and not get distracted."

Dad winked at me as Samuel left the room. For the rest of the day, my body twitched as I succumbed to the punishment that the M.E. Monster liked to inflict when I dared to enjoy myself but it was worth it.

CHAPTER THIRTY-SEVEN

My Other Family

Samuel asked me out that same night and I immediately said yes. It was strange but wonderful to think that I now had a boyfriend for the first time in my adult life. He made me feel so happy.

I received an email on the day I was due to travel up to King's College Hospital in London to have tests on my seizure activity done, that there was going to be a news story on that evening about my Pride of Britain nomination. I was already beginning to feel anxious, so I sent a text to Samuel and he immediately replied.

SAMUEL: *Oh my God! I'm so proud of you. That'll be the perfect way to introduce my family to you. I'll set the television to record and get them to watch it. Not many people can say that their girlfriend is on the news for a Pride of Britain shortlist!*

Funnily enough that did not settle any of my nerves. What would they think of the fact that their son was going out with a disabled girl who was pretty much bedbound? As if he could read my thoughts, my phone pinged with another message.

SAMUEL: *By the way Jessica, I can guarantee that they'll love you. Don't worry!*

Stewie had taken the day off to accompany Dad and me in the ambulance. Once we arrived at King's College Hospital, they pushed the ambulance trolley through the endless corridors. My eyes had to be covered by my dark glasses and I tried to look straight at the ceiling to stop the motion making me feel sick.

Another message from Samuel popped up on my mobile phone screen and Stewie saw my face light up.

"Right, can I just say that I'm amazing? How many years have you been asking me to find you a man? I had high hopes for that dating app but seeing you this happy makes me think I should give it a go too. Now I've helped you, it's your turn to be a hitch for me, got it?"

"I'll give it to you Stewie, going on that dating app was money well spent. Thank you! I'll take it upon myself to find you someone far quicker than it took you to help me." I laughed.

Whilst I was in hospital, I had the opportunity to go and visit some of the children that Share a Star had been helping. There were three children on the same ward who had all received multi-visceral transplants. When Dad and Stewie pushed the ambulance trolley in to see them, I felt overwhelmed. These kids were suffering so much and their screams could be heard from the corridor.

I went into the room of one of the children and the little boy sat in his bed quietly. His skin was tinged yellow and he had tubes giving him nutrition. My heart broke as I watched the nurses administer a list of medication into his body. I put out my hand and he held on to it. Even though the hand squeeze lasted about five minutes, I knew its effect would last an eternity for me.

After half an hour of seeing the children, I was pushed back to the ambulance to go home. It had been an emotional visit. Being able to visit those children had inspired me so much, but I was hit with the reality that the tests I had travelled up for were inconclusive. It must be down to the bastard M.E. Monster and it was just as Dr Nice had predicted—there was no treatment plan that would stop them.

Once we arrived home, the news was on in the living room and I was suddenly overcome with toe-curling nerves. Once the news went on to social media, I was inundated with messages of support flooding into my inbox. Again, the online community highlighted the very best parts of social media.

Share a Star was never about the accolades, it was simply helping make a small difference. The quote, *'Be the change that you wish to see in the world,'* spoke to me the moment I watched the news clip. To me, I hadn't done anything big, I had just done what I could, which changed the worlds of other families.

The finalists were doing far more incredible things in comparison to me, so it came as no surprise that I didn't win the overall award. The families who had nominated me couldn't hide their disappointment though.

A couple of weeks later, Dad came into my room juggling a parcel while filming me on his phone.

"It's for you." My puzzled expression made him laugh out loud. "Be careful, it's fragile!"

I opened the box and my jaw dropped at the sight of an

incredible glass award. I inspected it and saw that it did indeed have my name engraved on it. I pulled the award out of the box and saw a load of messages attached to it. As I flicked through them, there were messages of love from all of my online family.

"What does it say?" Dad asked.

"Dear Jessica, you were always the winner in my eyes. Thank you for all you do."

I was completely gobsmacked as I continued to read all the notes. For that moment, I felt like I was on cloud nine, surrounded by people who made my world a better place. As much as they felt I had helped them, they didn't realise quite how much they had helped me too.

CHAPTER THIRTY-EIGHT

Winter Wedding

My occupational health therapist and physio terrorist visited me a few days before we were due to leave for Tom and Jem's winter wedding in Hampshire. They made sure that everyone knew what the plan was—from how I needed to be lifted, as there was no hoist—to dealing with my fatigue.

"Promise me that you're going to take regular rests?" my occupational health therapist asked.

"Yes, I will definitely pace myself, no matter how excited I get!"

"So, you're bringing your carer, and I guess your boyfriend too?" she asked.

"Yes, he'll be there!" I grinned. I still couldn't believe I had a date for the wedding.

"Please make sure he or your carer are with you all the time—you know how quickly your health can deteriorate," my occupational health therapist said, as she looked at my physio terrorist, who nodded in agreement.

My physio terrorist smiled at me. "Enjoy it! This is a big moment. A lot of firsts will happen, and I can't wait to hear about them. Safe journey!"

I awoke early on the morning of the wedding to take a concoction of medication. The journey the day before had been exhausting; we had had to stop regularly because the motion made me feel nauseous. I had been told to take more pain relief to keep my symptoms at bay, as they were likely to flare up because of the adrenaline that was pumping through me.

After I was fed breakfast, my carer helped me get into my bridesmaid dress and steadied my hand, as I applied some makeup. Becky was getting ready with the other bridesmaids. There was a knock at the door and the hairdresser entered holding some GHD straighteners. She managed to do my hair whilst my head was propped up on a pillow. I had to remain flat for as long as possible to save my energy.

Once I was ready, Samuel changed into his suit.

"You definitely look quite dapper in a suit, Mr Bearman," I said.

"Why, thank you. I've never worn one before today," Samuel confessed.

"You should do it more. It's definitely a turn on!"

He grinned at me.

Mum entered my room looking glamorous in her outfit.

"Oh Sam, thank goodness you're here! It's a weight off my shoulders to know Jessica won't be on her own and has you."

He smiled and his cheeks went red. "Er... well... I'm glad I'm here with you all." Even though he knew my family now, Samuel was still shy in front of them.

Dad and Samuel had to lift me into my wheelchair together. They covered my face with a blanket to shield my eyes from the light. I met Becky and the other bridesmaids with a few minutes to spare before the wedding ceremony began.

Jem walked into the room with her dad. She looked absolutely stunning in her wedding dress. She grinned at me and bent down to hug me in my wheelchair. "I'm so glad you made it!" She turned to Dad who was pushing my wheelchair. "It looks like you're going to be a bridesmaid too, Colin!"

As Samuel and I listened to Ed Sheeran's *Thinking Out Loud* playing in the background, I knew I that I was missing out on seeing Tom and Jem's first dance. It had been an incredible day and I had achieved far more than anyone had imagined I would. The ceremony had gone seamlessly and I had even managed to stand up for a few seconds for the official wedding photos. I had shown Samuel off to relatives and family friends that I hadn't seen since becoming unwell.

But I didn't want to miss the dance, even though I could feel that my adrenaline would not last much longer.

Samuel looked at me. "Do you want to go back and watch them dance? It's a once in a lifetime moment."

For a second, I thought of the payback the M.E. Monster would surely give me but the thought of seeing Tom and Jem dance was too tempting. We rang Stewie, who was drunk, and he and Samuel managed to pick me up.

Stewie left my reclined wheelchair on the dance floor and disappeared to find Tom and Jem. Tom came and knelt by my chair. He gave me a cuddle.

"I wanted to see your first dance," I whispered in his ear.

"I'm glad," Tom said before he whisked me up into the air.

The guests all whooped with joy as his 6'4 frame whirled me around to the music. Jem joined us and we had a moment together dancing to *Let it Go* from *Frozen*. Granted, it was a terrible song choice, but I didn't care. I managed to celebrate their special day with them. I had achieved the goal that I had dreamed of for years.

The journey home from the wedding knocked me for six. I spent the next few days in a trance, trying to recover. Samuel stayed with me at the wedding venue, but he had to go back to his work, as a sales assistant in Essex, while we returned to Kent.

It was just before Samuel's birthday, so I asked Becky to arrange a pre-birthday celebration just before she was flying out to Austria to visit her best friend. She helped me decorate my room with balloons and made an allergen-free birthday cake that was 'Jessica-friendly.'

Afterwards Samuel laid next to me looking up at the ceiling. I put my cold hands over his eyes, which made him jump.

"What the. . . ?"

"I've got one last birthday present for you!"

"Now what would that be?"

"Where in the world would you like to go? Pick anywhere!"

Samuel was silent for a moment. "I love New Zealand."

"I'm going to take you on a romantic getaway then."

He looked bemused. "Dare I ask how?"

"My room can take me anywhere in the world," I explained. "I can go from Scotland to Australia in a day."

"Well that's certainly a cheaper way of travelling." He laughed.

"Are you ready?" He nodded. "So I think that we should visit the places that Lord of the Rings was filmed first. I mean the scenery in that film was just incredible."

"It sure was!"

"We're standing at the top of the mountain where Gandalf

came charging down as the white wizard at the end of the Twin Towers. The sun is shining brightly across the bright blue skies. The golden light touches everything as far as the eye can see, from the streams to the snow on the top of the mountains. There are so many different colours, from green hills to wildflower. . ."

The exhaustion began to take over, as the pain of the M.E. Monster tormented me my fragile body.

"No matter what way you travel, you still get travel sickness," I mumbled before falling asleep.

"Thank you for the best birthday present," he whispered in my ear.

CHAPTER THIRTY-NINE

Love Is Pain

The next day was a blur, I was too fatigued to think and the pain in every part of my body was excruciating. Samuel was back in Essex, Becky was at the airport and I was alone.

By the time my carer had gone home I began to feel unwell. It started with a dull ache in my stomach but an hour later the pain had changed, and it felt like I was being stabbed. I managed to call my parents into my room just before I was violently sick. I prayed it was just a one-off, but the sickness kept coming long into the night. By the early hours of the morning, I had been sick over a dozen times.

Mum paced the room, wracking her brains as to what could possibly be making me this unwell.

"What did you have to eat today?" Mum asked whilst Dad soothed me.

"I don't know," I blearily replied before throwing up again. "Something with rice."

"Was it piping hot?" Mum asked urgently.

"I. . . I don't know," I murmured as I wretched into the bowl Dad was holding tightly.

"You know that rice needs to be piping hot to prevent food poisoning darling. Tell me that it was?"

I felt so stupid because I couldn't remember. The M.E. Monster had been callously tormenting me ever since I had returned from the wedding. I spent the whole day drifting in and out of consciousness and my words had slurred anytime I tried to talk.

"Dunno. . . I. . . just. . . don't. . . know."

"How could you not know?" Mum snapped.

The M.E. Monster sent agony into every part of my aching exhausted body. I tried so hard to recall what I had eaten in a semi-conscious state.

"I can't. . . remember. . . it." I threw up again. "I can't remember it being piping hot."

I groaned as I tried to grasp hold of the bowl again.

"If it's food poisoning, I'll be so angry. Rice, for goodness sake! That's why we have carers, to look after her, not to have this happen!" Mum exclaimed.

"Hang on, let us see if it calms down and I'll call the night doctor," Dad gently said.

But it didn't and within an hour they were both convinced it was food poisoning. Mum sat with me all night, as I became more and more poorly. I couldn't keep any fluids down, let alone eat anything. I had important medication that needed to be in my system to control the symptoms that the M.E. Monster caused. Not being able to keep medications down was dangerous for me.

I desperately wanted to feel the comfort of Samuel holding me in his arms, but I didn't want him to see me like this. *Maybe I should text him?* I fumbled with my phone, desperately trying to press the buttons but I didn't even have the cognitive energy to put a sentence together. A tear of frustration left my eye, and Mum stroked my face. She took the phone off me. "Don't worry. I've let Samuel know, darling. Rest."

I groggily woke up the next day. My body ached, my chest was tight and I felt weak. The antiemetic medication that the doctor had given in the early hours of the morning hadn't stopped my sickness, so the only option was for me to be taken into hospital via ambulance. I loathed this bloody disease.

Mum came quietly into the room and stood by my bed.

"Look who I've got with me."

I turned my head and tried to focus. *Samuel?* As soon as his hand touched mine, I knew it was him. A mixture of emotions filled me; I was relieved to see him but I was terrified of him seeing me in this way. I hadn't shown him this part of the M.E. Monster; my fear of scaring him off was far too great. I didn't want him to have to be taken through all this when we'd only been dating for three months. But as he sat next to me, I knew that I not only wanted him with me, I needed him too.

Mum came into my room talking on video call to someone. My heart let out a sigh of relief because I recognised my sister's voice.

"It had to be whilst I was away, didn't it? Well, Samuel will have to be there in my place. He's a good guy, so I know he'll look after her well. Be impressed, I've actually been using my phone to text him."

"That's a miracle in itself baby because you're abysmal at texting!" Mum responded.

Hearing Becky's voice made me feel calmer. Samuel stroked my head as I continued to vomit. Stupid, poxy chronic ill health.

The ambulance came, at which point my body was so weakened I could barely whisper a sound. My head was pounding. Samuel accompanied me and kept moving my hair out of my face, as the bumps in the road made me vomit.

As soon as I got there, the nurses tried to find my veins to give me fluids to hydrate me. They tried everywhere until the consultant finally managed to get one in. They took my blood, swabbed me and then checked my observations, whilst I continued to be sick over and over again.

Yet still Samuel sat there until the early hours of the morning, holding my hand. My dad joined him and passed him a cup of tea.

"I can take over if you want a break, Samuel."

"Thanks, but I'm fine. I'd rather be with her."

The hours ticked by as we waited for the results to determine what was wrong. They stayed with me until I was moved on to the ward. The nurses had decorated the ward for Christmas, which was a week away. I desperately wanted to be at home for my first Christmas with Samuel.

"Ring me if you need me, I'll be up at any time for you, Jessica. Love you," Samuel whispered to me.

If I had any more energy, I would have called back for him to stay with me.

I couldn't sleep. The noises were excruciating for my hypersensitive ears and the lights burnt my eyes. It was all too easy to just ring Samuel, but I knew he needed rest too. The pain became immeasurable from the M.E., let alone the stomach stabbing. My mind began to trick me with horrific thoughts. *Maybe something else was wrong with me? Maybe nothing was wrong with me?*

After years of torment from people playing with my mind, I found the smallest questions panicked me.

"It's all in your head."

"More excuses."

"I'd love to be in bed like you, getting all that attention."

The list was endless. I knew it was all rubbish but when I was vulnerable, it niggled at the back of my mind. I fell into a dazed sleep, where I dreamed of fighting consultants, because the M.E. Monster could attack at any time.

In the morning Samuel came back on to the ward with my carer. I could tell that he had barely got any sleep by the look on his face. The doctors confirmed that they were dealing with gastritis due to food poisoning. They had to run a few checks and needed to keep me in until I stopped being sick. Samuel stayed by my side all day. He hadn't ever seen someone other than me be really unwell, so it was an unpleasant shock to his system.

Everything else could wait. His priority was me and that was the greatest comfort. He held my hand tightly and sat there silently. He wasn't talking to me about how he was feeling, but he spent the time I was resting sending messages to his family. My only hope was that they were giving him the emotional support that, at that precise moment, I couldn't offer.

I knew I was awful company. I was exhausted, stressed and in a place full of stimulation. It wasn't a good environment for anyone, let alone someone who had to live with the M.E. Monster inside of them. My body felt like every cell was screaming in pain. I was cross with myself that I hadn't realised that the food that caused this wasn't cooked enough.

It seemed like I was far away from the celebrations of Tom

and Jem's wedding. I had managed so many firsts there, so many triumphs but now we were back to square one—a hospital room.

I focused on breathing slowly and deeply to calm down. I wasn't well enough to be frustrated too. That was exhausting in itself. Although Samuel was scared stiff, he remained by my side. I didn't want him to see me when I was completely dependent on others. I didn't want him to have to help roll me on to a bedpan because I didn't have the energy to do it myself.

The M.E. Monster stripped me of all dignity, and I cursed it as I relied on Samuel's help. Yet, Samuel didn't budge. He wasn't scared away by my suffering. In fact, it was bringing us closer together.

I had always said that I suffered from an exhaustion that hurt, but it was only now that I realised that love hurts too. It hurts to see those we love suffer; in fact the pain was even more difficult to explain when love had anything to do with it.

As the day turned into night, Samuel said, "Jessica, I know you're suffering but I need you to know that I'm not going anywhere. I love you and I can't find the words to tell you how much you mean to me. I'm here for the long haul."

I broke down in tears. For years, I felt like I was navigating this journey alone. I wasn't alone anymore. I had someone to share the suffering with. I didn't need to do it on my own and it was okay to not always feel positive when everything went wrong.

Even though I barely had the energy to move, I squeezed my hand around Samuel's hand, so he knew how much I loved him.

CHAPTER FORTY

The C Bomb

It always perplexed me that I managed to cope so well with being an inpatient for over four years continuously. I'd only been in for three days and was already struggling. All the sensory overload made me feel agitated and exhausted. To keep sane, I began to dream of my escape. It was Christmas time and the last place that I wanted to be was the hospital. I was going to do everything in my power to get home in time for Christmas.

"Your mum's a nurse, isn't she?" a junior doctor asked before ward round began. "Oh, and your dad's a paramedic? So you'll be able to have medications?"

"My mum could give me any intramuscular injections of antiemetics that I need, if that would help?"

Mum and Dad were both such crucial parts of my life and my care more than ever. They got me out of hospital early because they were capable of nursing me with their own medical knowledge. It seemed strange, but to be in hospital for short periods more often was more difficult for my body and the rest of my family to adjust to. Now with Samuel and Becky's new boyfriend Ben in the equation, my family was growing, and it was essential that their wellbeing was thought of in all decisions I made.

"We'll wait for the results of the blood test and then we'll get you home on injections so you can be there for Christmas," the consultant said.

Overjoyed, I rang Mum, but she didn't answer. She texted and said she was just coming in. Mum looked troubled when she entered, but still smiled when she saw me. After telling her everything, she held my hand.

"Baby, I just wondered if there was a chance you could come home tomorrow? I've got something planned on the day they're looking to discharge you."

Planned?

"It's just typical, but basically I've found a lump in my boob," Mum continued.

"What?" I whispered.

"It's really fine," Mum said quickly. "It's just annoying that it's now, especially around Christmas. I don't want you worrying. We've got to get you better. It's probably just a cyst but you know what they're like, it must be checked."

I had a lump in my breast years ago and it wasn't anything sinister. Cancer doesn't run in my family.

As soon as she left, I spoke to my consultant who agreed that I could return home the next day with extra medication that my parents could administer until I had built my strength back up. Despite the nurse's concern that it was too early for me to be discharged, I knew it was the right decision for me and my family. That was all that mattered.

In the morning Samuel packed all my belongings, ready for

the ambulance to take me home. I was nervous about the mammogram Mum was going to have, on top of having to look after me. Even though the effects of the food poisoning would ease, the doctors believed that the overreaction of the M.E. Monster's response to it would take longer to recover from.

I was reliant on constant antiemetic injections to control the sickness. My body was weak from the constant stimuli on the hospital ward. Not only the bright lights, but noises and people talking all the time. It never stopped and I had lost my spoons of energy, just through the sensory overload.

Dad and Kip couldn't pick me up. They were both working overtime and hadn't been able to take time off. The reality of the overstretched ambulance service meant we could be waiting anywhere from four to ten hours. Living on a constant adrenaline rush was damaging to my health. I couldn't rest might leave at any moment, but I didn't have the energy to be constantly on the go.

Samuel could see that I was starting to get agitated, so he sat by my side and we spoke about the plans for Christmas. I was looking forward to being able to spend my first Christmas with him. We'd been together for three months, but I was not used to having someone to share my life with.

"Now, can you guess what I have got you for Christmas? It's something special that I think you'll like."

My face fell. With all the stress and this hospital admission, I hadn't bought Samuel something for Christmas! With four days to go and no energy, I didn't know how on earth I was going to be able to do anything about it.

"I'm so sorry, Samuel. I'm not going to have time to get you something."

"Don't be silly! My Christmas present is being able to get you home and be with you."

I managed to squeeze his hand tightly. I appreciated him more than he could ever know.

Finally, the ambulance crew arrived to take us home at 11:30pm. Samuel was asleep on the chair, and I was staring into an abyss, thinking of all the uncertainties that I faced. *What if there was something more to Mum's lump? How would I cope at home?* I didn't want to be a failed discharge—one that leaves hospital, only to return a day later. I didn't have the strength nor the energy.

When I got home, I forgot all my fears of what the results of Mum's tests would be. I was occupied with my own health. I had to make sure I survived each moment, minute by minute, hour after hour.

Christmas came and went. I spent the day with Samuel, curled up in my bed, as my energy levels were low. Becky came home for Christmas and demanded that we all dress up in the tackiest Christmas accessories she could find. The payback from the wedding, my admission, and then Christmas was horrible. The New Year had to bring some better health for me.

Mum was more anxious than ever as she waited for the results of her scan. *Why hadn't she heard yet?*

On New Year's Eve, she came into my room where I was hanging out with Samuel. Her eyes darted to the door, as she beckoned Becky and her boyfriend Ben in.

"I'm bringing you all together because I need you to know, I mean, I told Dad before he went to work." She looked at me then at Becky. "I've got breast cancer. And it's stage four."

I looked at Becky whose face was set in stone. Her eyes didn't move as she looked straight ahead.

"I'm so sorry. I'm starting treatment and I've been put on a high dose of a drug that will help. We will, we will," her voice broke on the last word.

"Do this together." Becky finished quietly, as Ben squeezed her shoulder.

Mum looked like a startled rabbit staring into the headlights and Becky hugged her tightly.

"I need us to make this New Year the most fun we've had, because we have had fun, haven't we? Real fun. And I don't want it to stop. It can't because that's how I'm going to beat this bastard disease," Mum said.

It took all my effort to smile and tell her it would be okay.

After the door shut, my world crashed in. The exhaustion seeped through my veins, then adrenaline pummelled me, so I became short of breath. I began to cry, completely oblivious to Samuel holding me.

I let myself fall into him and yelled out loud, letting all the pain out. I curled into a ball and Samuel just held me tightly.

My mum had always been one of my rocks. I wasn't stupid, there was no stage five. I tried to exhale some air from my exhausted lungs but the M.E. Monster cackled and tortured me for even daring to feel.

2016

CHAPTER FORTY-ONE

Yin And Yang

Mum's cancer diagnosis made me revaluate my life. My relationship with Samuel was serious and we were a pillar of strength for each other. Although we were different, we seemed to complement each other perfectly, like yin and yang.

Samuel wanted to look after me properly, so he learnt how to give me my medication and deal with my seizures. He was already becoming a pro at being able to look after me when I crash because of the M.E. Monster.

Having him support me helped take the pressure off my family, who were struggling to cope in their own ways. Dad didn't want to show us how broken he was about Mum's health, so he threw himself into work.

Mum was very private about her suffering. For as long as I could remember, she suffered from bipolar disorder. She felt like she had no control over her life, especially when she got cancer. She was fixated on dealing with everything in her own way, which was to keep it secret from family and friends but this became hard for the rest of us because we couldn't talk to anyone. Tom found it the hardest to deal with. He was used to our family constantly going through medical dramas but they were always because of my health, not Mum's too. How much more could honestly be thrown at us?

Becky kept herself busy. She was never one to talk about how she was feeling. She was too used to looking after everyone else to acknowledge what she was going through.

And me? I just felt lost. I was always the polar opposite of Becky: my coping mechanism was to talk about my feelings. I confided my deepest fears to Samuel which helped me and thankfully Samuel's family was an emotional support for him.

For days I had been occupied by my inner thoughts. I kept looking at the picture on my bedside table of Gran with her twinkling eyes and smile that lit up the room. She would have known what to say to Mum. She would have comforted us all and reminded us that life could indeed be, in her words, 'mouldy.' Gran would have loved Samuel. I remember her drilling the importance of being happy into me and Becky from a young age.

"Happiness is everything, you two. Don't sacrifice it for someone else because you deserve to live your best life. Do you hear me, girls?

"Yes Gran, I'll only settle for a house full of chocolate!" Becky had exclaimed.

"Well, that's not quite what I meant, but you have the right idea."

Samuel was my happiness and I needed him.

"Jessica, I'm not sure what you think of this idea," Samuel said to me a week after Mum's bombshell. "But I want to be here for you all the time. I know this has been a whirlwind relationship, but I don't want you to have to face this journey on your own." Samuel cuddled into me.

"I want you to be here too. I need you."

"What do you say to us moving in together? Obviously, with the permission of your parents," Samuel said.

I wasn't expecting that. "But what about your family? And your work?"

"My family love you and want me to support you. And work is work. I'll find another job in Kent."

I hadn't felt this happy in ages! "That'd be amazing. I'd like that"

We kissed and I felt as though the weight of the world had been taken off my shoulders. I wouldn't feel alone anymore.

Everything that I had been through in the past decade got on top of me. I was haunted by my past and traumatised by the abuse I suffered from Jackson in hospital. In the past, if something happened, I put to the back of my mind. I dealt with Jackson by changing my name from Jess to Jessica and making a fresh new start.

I was now the closest that I had ever been to a man and I was so happy. So why did Jackson get in my thoughts?

"But who'd listen to you, Jess?" His words taunt me.

I told Samuel about Jackson early on in our relationship, but I felt embarrassed to tell him that I was thinking of him again. At first it was just the odd thought, then he came into my dreams and I then I got nightmares. I wake up breathing fast, drenched in my own cold sweat.

Having Samuel live with me felt completely natural. He fitted so well into my family and he became my main carer overnight. Although our relationship grew stronger by the day, I had started to notice that he wasn't quite himself.

In the night I would wake up to him thrashing around in the bed, desperately calling,

"Jessica! Jessica! I need you!"

I slept in a hospital bed, we'd got a put-me-up bed for Samuel that connected to mine. I tried to make him stir by speaking to him and he woke up panting for breath. Sometimes he was half-asleep and he murmured for me not to leave him, before turning over and going back to sleep.

After a bad nightmare, Samuel woke me up.

"You see him, don't you?"

"Who?" I asked, playing for time.

"That excuse-for-a-man Jackson."

I felt sick. "How do you know?"

"I hear you screaming his name in your sleep."

"I'm getting flashbacks of him but I don't know why. I didn't tell you because. . . well. . . I didn't want to scare you off."

"Jessica, you know I love you for you and everything that comes with it. You can't scare me off." Samuel hugged me tight.

I cuddled into his neck. "And your nightmares?" I could feel him stiffen. "What are they about?"

He sighed. "Losing you. I can't bear the thought of it. It was hard seeing you in that ill in hospital. Every time you crash from the Monster, I just panic."

I had no idea Samuel's bad dreams were about me. As the days went by my health continued to fluctuate with multiple seizures and crashes from the M.E. Monster. Samuel's anxiety worsened. He started to have debilitating panic attacks before work that would glue him to the spot. His irrational fear of the unknown paralysed him.

It was horrendous to watch the living hell that his anxiety caused every day.

Becky had to drive Mum to and from her radiotherapy sessions three times a week. The cancer didn't make Mum look ill, but the treatment made her terribly sick and pale.

Overnight, she went from being the life and soul of the party to a shadow of herself. The day before the radiotherapy, she was darting around running errands. After it there was a stark contrast, as she was pushed around in a wheelchair. By the time she recovered from the treatment, it was time for the next cycle.

The stress of living with so many struggling people in one house was phenomenal. Whilst Mum was suffering in her bed, Samuel started on medication for his depression. Becky was being treated for bipolar too. I was painfully working through my past trauma with a counsellor, which made me emotional. Dad would come home after working long hours, and snap at everyone. It felt at times like everyone was falling apart.

The only silver lining to Mum's health battles was that we all understood how important it was to live in the moment. Despite the odds, my relationship with Samuel went from strength to strength. I felt his complete devotion to me and I couldn't imagine being without him. Our lives had taken so many twists and turns in the five months we'd been together.

We found joy in the simple things, like going for a walk in the sunshine with me in my wheelchair. I knew I wanted to be with him for the rest of my life, and I knew he felt the same.

CHAPTER FORTY-TWO

A Day To Remember

My needs increased over the month since Mum started her treatment and my carer had to spend every hour of the day with me to keep me stable. Samuel and I yearn to have some more quality time together on our own, like a normal relationship. Dreaming became our escapism, as we spent the evenings talking about what we wanted together in the future.

I knew Samuel was up to something when he started spending more time with Becky. They would talk in hushed voices and Becky started opening up to me about what she wished would happen in her relationship with Ben.

"I wish he lived with me like Samuel does with you. Would you want to get married at all? I would."

"I would love to get married one day, but I'm sure I'll be waiting a while. I have to keep pinching myself that he's a part of my crazy life," I said.

"You never know. It's been so lovely to see you so content with him. You make a dream team."

"I'm pretty darn lucky."

"He's lucky to have you too."

The next morning I heard the phone ringing in my sleep,

but I couldn't focus on where it was coming from. I always found mornings intensely challenging due to my health. I viewed the world through frosted glass at that time. I have to go through hours of chronic nausea and confusion, before I come to a conscious state.

I could hear a voice talking to me. *Samuel?*

"Jessica, your carer is off sick today, so are you happy with me looking after you on my own?"

I nodded slowly.

"Just no medical emergencies today!"

After I had my medication, I was enjoying the fact that we had time together on our own. We were watching a film when suddenly Samuel stood up and put the television on pause. He bent over like he had dropped something on the floor, but he had my bed control, and the bed was moving to the ground. I look at him quizzically.

What was he picking up from the ground?

I put some weight into my arms to lift my body, so I could see what he was doing.

There he was, knelt on the floor, holding a ring in his hand.

Was I dreaming? I stared at him with my eyes wide.

"Will you marry me, Jessica?"

I couldn't believe the words had come out of his mouth. He wanted to be with me for the rest of his life in sickness and health. As my brain tried to comprehend what had just happened, I suddenly realised that I hadn't answered him. My shock turned into a smile and I raised my hands to my mouth, before shouting, "Yes!"

Throughout my time suffering with the M.E. Monster and being unable to communicate, I had taken it upon myself to dream of my future. I had planned the colour theme for my wedding, where I would work, and what countries I would travel to. As a teen I had a childlike naivety; I believed that anything could happen.

As the years went on, nothing had changed and even with the most positive outlook, my hope for everything that I wanted from life dwindled. My life expectations changed and I didn't expect anyone to want to live a life in one room with me and my limitations but look at me now. I was going to be someone's wife!

As I felt the ring on my finger, I grinned and did a happy excited dance in my bed. It was the best feeling in the entire world but the M.E. Monster zapped me of all my energy to remind me that he was still in charge.

Once the news of our engagement broke on social media our phones kept pinging with notifications from people all over the world congratulating us. The idea of planning a wedding around the M.E. Monster was challenging, but exciting because I was doing it with my best friend.

I woke Samuel up in the middle of the night, when I got wild ideas of how we could make our wedding the most perfect day. I thought of colour themes, guest lists and song choices.

Whenever I thought about the style of dress that I wanted to wear I just couldn't imagine how I would get down the aisle. Even though my wheelchair gave me a new-found freedom, my dream was to walk down the aisle on my wedding day.

My life had been full of constant suffering and boundaries that the M.E. Monster made, but I wanted our day to be about Samuel and me. Despite everything I had faced in my life, I didn't want the Monster to have a say on what I could do at my wedding.

As Dr Nice said multiple times, "You don't like accepting that your life is different to that of your friends."

Dates and numbers were always important to me. I loved adding intricate details to special occasions personal to me and my loved ones.

What would be the most memorable date for our wedding?

As I scrolled through dates on my phone's calendar, I realised that the 29th April—which would have been my Gran's seventy-seventh birthday—was going to be on a Saturday next year. I excitedly showed my phone to Samuel and he grinned because he knew how important my gran was to me.

"Looks like we've got a date Jessica!"

Mum was struggling. Watching her go through treatment every other day for weeks at a time was hard. She was waiting to have a scan done to see whether the treatment had stopped the cancer from spreading and shrunk any of the tumours.

In a way, she now understood the suffering I had been facing for years. The exhaustion after every treatment confined her to her bed. She was continuously nauseous and her skin felt like it was on fire with electrical currents. I hated seeing her suffer so terribly, knowing there was nothing I could do to help.

I tried to keep her mind occupied by talking about the plans for the wedding. Looking at different wedding themes and ideas on Pinterest took her mind away from her suffering. She lost a lot of weight from the radiotherapy and her mental health was all over the place. The medication she took for her bipolar had stopped working due to the other medication she was on for the cancer.

The Share a Star team were planning our most ambitious fundraiser yet: an evening ball for all our supporters that I was hoping to attend. Mum's suffering made me fully understand how helpless the families of the children from Share a Star felt.

My own experience with living in hospital as a teenager had hugely influenced my ideas for Share a Star. I often came up with new plans in the middle of the night, when I was in too much pain to move. There was always somebody worse off. Whilst I was lying in agony, another family was dealing with the death of their child. I knew this was the reality of suffering.

If I could make a surprise entrance to the ball to thank all the people helping raise vital funds to continue to help more families, then I was going to do it.

After we got engaged, the postman excitedly knocked on the door to deliver a letter.

"It's not often I deliver letters from 10 Downing Street."

Samuel saw the embossed stamp in the corner of the envelope. His mouth dropped, as he read the name of the recipient.

"Jessica, can I open this?" he asked.

"You aren't normally bothered about my post!"

"I am about this little beauty." He pointed at the crisp envelope in his hands. He rubbed his fingers over the printed envelope and brought it closer so I could read what it said.

"The Prime Minister?" I gasped. "What would he want with me?"

"I have no idea, but I want to see it! Maybe, he's just

congratulating us on our engagement? I'd better check," he teased, as he moved the letter out of my reach.

Once I had grabbed the envelope, I carefully tore it open to see a letter from none other than Prime Minister David Cameron. I read the words over and over again. I had won a Points of Light Award.

We found the press release about my story on the internet with this quote from David Cameron.

With Share a Star, Jessica has shown a remarkable commitment to supporting other young people who face serious ill health or have very ill siblings. The peer support and family trips she organises have brought much-needed joy to hundreds of severely unwell young people and their families, despite her own ill health. To those who have received her kindness and empathy she is a true point of light.

I had just won a National Award for my charity work! I was not a particular fan of the government, but a letter of recognition was a welcome treat. It was incredible to think that even from one room where I was isolated from the rest of the world, I had managed to be noticed.

The Points of Lights Award was a government initiative to praise those making a difference in their communities. There was a person awarded with the Points of Light Award every day.

I went on to Twitter to share the news, and shockingly found that I was being followed by none other than *the* Prime Minister's Twitter account! *What?* I hoped that the awareness would bring much needed support to the work that my volunteers and I were trying to do.

When I thought of how much Becky had suffered from

seeing me so poorly from such an impressionable age, it broke my heart. She had lost time with my parents, as she was moved between different places, whilst they acted as superheroes keeping everything afloat. The scenes she saw in the hospital scarred her for life. The tubes that were connected to my motionless body haunted her. Our story was just one example of why supporting the whole family was important.

Not only was the ball going to be the first time that I'd been out for the evening since I was fourteen, but it would be a good chance to assess how I would manage an event like our wedding!

CHAPTER FORTY-THREE

The Ball

I always had to wear industrial ear plugs due to the M.E. Monster. Sound caused me physical pain and made me feel sick. The Monster would take any noise and amplify it, until it was unbearable. At the beginning of my journey, I was unable to cope with the sound of my dad's voice, even when he whispered. Even though it had vastly improved, I was still used to the stillness of my four walls and trying to concentrate on lots of people zapped me of all my energy quickly.

To get to the ball, I not only needed to be able to be sat in my wheelchair for a lot longer than I was used to but I needed to cope with the motion of being moved in it too. I was preparing myself for the stimulation by going on rides around the village with Samuel and Mum. It was always nice to be free from the house I'd been imprisoned in for more years than I could remember. After all these years, I still knew the route by heart from being a child. When we passed the horses in the field, they would canter alongside my wheelchair, as if they remembered me. It felt like a blissful escape from my isolated existence.

The plan for our wedding was always at the back of mind.

When my physio terrorist and occupational health therapist came to see me together, I discussed whether my idea of walking down the aisle was possible.

The physio terrorist gulped at my proposition. "I mean, to get you physically down the aisle in one piece is probably the biggest challenge I've ever worked on with you, or anybody for that matter."

"It's not just physically, I need to work with you so you could cognitively deal with all the stimulation without crashing," the occupational health therapist weighed in. "It's a big ask, Jessica. We would have to work *with* your body."

"We did think that getting you to your brother's wedding was a big ask though so it's definitely possible," the physio terrorist said. "I think our main problem will be getting you used to the physiology of standing, because currently your pulse rockets and your blood pressure drops."

"The joys of having a messed up autonomic system." I sighed.

"Try the ball first, see how you manage that and we'll make a plan from then on," the occupational health therapist said.

"Just don't push your body," the physio terrorist added. "We don't need you crashing. We have just over a year until your big day and you know what? A lot can happen in a year."

If it was going to be at all possible, then I knew that my team would make it happen. They were both experts in working with what my body could manage, which sometimes felt like it was at a snail's pace. Their understanding of how the M.E. Monster affected me, would give me the best possible chance of success.

In order to help my body manage the ball, I regimented my days strictly between rest and short activities. There were so many things that I wanted to be able to do that I needed to break it down. Although my symptoms often incapacitated me, my mind was as free as a butterfly to hope and dream.

As my excitement for the ball mounted, I spent hours scouring the internet with Becky to shop for the perfect dress. I wanted it to be a classic, floor-length, ball gown, but practical enough for me to wear in my wheelchair.

We scrawled through pages of different styles and Blissy joined in from afar by sending pictures of various dresses to us both via Facebook. We found the perfect one and bought it. I knew I was going to feel like a princess on the day. The dress was long, dusky purple and bedecked with jewels.

When it arrived in the post and I saw it, my jaw dropped; it was even more beautiful than I imagined it would be. As soon as Becky helped me try it on I felt like a million dollars. For the first time in my life I felt beautiful and confident. I was ready to go to the ball.

On the day of the ball, Samuel and Dad went to the venue early to make sure everything was ready. Mum, Becky and I got glammed up together. It was the first time that I had spent quality time doing girly things with Mum and Becky since I was a teenager. Even then, we didn't hang out loads. I was mean and moody, and Becky was a stroppy ten-year-old. Even at Tom and Jem's wedding, Becky was with the other bridesmaids and I was with my carer.

Becky helped Mum step into her sparkling dress, and grinned as she did the zip up.

"Et voila! You look stunning, Mum. You'll be the belle of the ball."

Mum swirled around in a circle to flaunt her dress. If I didn't know about the evil disease attacking her body, I would never know she was ill. Her face lit up. She was looking better because she was having a break from treatment for two weeks. The radiotherapy happened in cycles: three weeks of treatment and then two weeks rest.

Mum zipped up Becky's dress and when she turned around, I gasped. The classic emerald coloured dress fitted her like a glove and flaunted her incredible figure.

"Why thank you!" Becky beamed. "Just recycling an old bridesmaid dress."

It was my turn next. Becky slipped the floaty ball gown dress on me as I laid on my bed. I had never dressed up like that before, but as the dress zipped up, I exuded a self-confidence I didn't normally possess. I stood up for a few seconds, with Mum and Becky holding me up. The three of us looked at each other, taking in the fact that we were getting ready to go out together for the first time since I had become unwell.

Mum hugged us both. Despite the uncertainty of whether I would manage to go 'out-out,' I was now ready to go to the ball.

It was pitch black as we got close to the venue. As we entered there was a hubbub of people coming and going in every direction. I tried to focus on those around me, but I felt like a startled rabbit in bright headlights. I saw Stewie and Tom in the crowd, looking dapper in their black-tie suits. Jem was next to Tom, looking glamorous with her sister. They came over and helped to make sure I was in a comfortable position in my recliner wheelchair.

A sea of purple and gold balloons filled the room where the function was being held. Everyone was silent as Dad announced that I had arrived and invited me to the stage. My stomach was somersaulting as Samuel pushed my wheelchair to the front of the room where I gave my speech about the importance of giving back.

The applause rang through my ears, and I had to take a moment to adjust the earplugs to drown out some of the noise. I was inundated with people coming up to me afterwards to congratulate me on my speech and tell me how I had inspired them.

I stayed for as long as I possibly could which included parts of the auction. I had done a painting for the occasion and I want to make sure it raised a fair amount of money for Share a Star, but I had to leave before I heard the winner.

I passed a drunken Stewie on my way out and made him promise to put down a good price for it. When I reached the car with Samuel, ready for Mum to drive us home, I questioned whether Stewie actually realised what he had agreed to. . . I guessed he'd soon find out!

The pain crept through my body, as we drove home. I cried out, as I felt each bump in the road. We arrived home and Samuel moved the wheelchair out of the car. He was perfectly capable of looking after me alone, so Mum helped to me get out before she went back to the ball.

In my speech, I mentioned the young people who were no longer with us. In my eyes, they're the stars watching over us at night. As Samuel fiddled with the lock on the back door, I looked up to see millions of stars sparkling in the night skies. I believed that one of them was my Gran, because she loved a bit of sparkle more than anything.

I stared up at the stars and imagined which one was her and what stars the young people had chosen. The stars were watching and cheering me on as I was taken inside by my fiancé. My first night out-out from the confines of my house would always be one to remember.

CHAPTER FORTY-FOUR

Millions Missing

Ever since I became unwell with M.E. I had been missing from the life I should have been living. I should have graduated from university, travelled the world with my friends like we always said we would do. It was ten years of suffering, a whole decade, 3,650 days.

Social media was both a blessing and a curse to me. Whilst I had connected with many other M.E. sufferers by using it, I also had to watch my school friends living their lives to the fullest, without being able to join in.

The scary reality was I was just one of *millions* of sufferers, who were missing from their lives too. The daily suffering was exhausting, as was the isolation. We needed to be heard and desperately needed to be seen too. When I did my awareness video in 2012 I tried to make my suffering visible but I didn't expect to still be explaining it four years later. We deserved better than this.

There was an underworld of M.E. sufferers who had started to fight the everyday ignorance that we face, by sharing their stories. There were news articles in local and national papers, television interviews and even documentaries being made.

For the past three years, I had been quietly filming all parts of my life for an American documentary called *Unrest*, to show the devastating effects of this disease. It had involved a camera crew coming to my house as well as being interviewed over the internet. I finished recording it last summer, and it was in the editing process. Nobody could contemplate that I didn't even possess the energy to wash myself. It seemed unbelievable that I hadn't been well enough to have a shower since I was fifteen.

The exhaustion that I felt daily, physically hurt every muscle in my body. There were no days off or holidays. The Monster was callous and stripped me of my dignity. No one saw the demoralising crashes that I suffer from. I couldn't even roll myself on to a bedpan.

When I had first become hospitalised, I believed whole-heartedly that I would fully recover. I hadn't even contemplated that I would still be suffering with it a decade later. For many years, I fought it. I always believed in a Disney-style fairy-tale ending of living happily ever after. In that dream I believed that the M.E. Monster would get driven away. Whilst there was no biomedical treatment for M.E. I knew that the only way forwards was to co-exist with it.

It wasn't just me that I wanted to live for. I was getting ready to start a new life with Samuel. I potentially had limited time with Mum, and I didn't want the majority of my memories of being back in my family home to be in a darkened room, shut away from the world. Samuel was teaching me to live and experience life, instead of just surviving.

There was a demonstration being held as part of M.E. Awareness Week, in cities all over the world. It was called Millions Missing and M.E. sufferers were joining forces to create a global protest in major cities. The fact that M.E. sufferers, who were often mainly housebound, were risking their health by taking to the streets to represent all of us highlighted how desperate we were to find a treatment that could help us get better.

Some of the people going were patients, and loved ones were planning to travel in the place of those too ill to get there. I was going to attend it via the internet, because the trip to London was too far for me to manage. The plan was to stun the public with a visual interpretation of how many millions of people are missing. A pair of shoes would be placed on the streets for every M.E. sufferer missing from society. Each pair had a tag attached, with the name of the person who was not there to represent themselves.

I chose a pair of Converse trainers that were brown with red laces. I always loved those shoes; they reminded me of when I was fifteen and I had tried to convince my parents to get me a pair for my birthday. Even though I couldn't wear them often, I asked for new clothes and shoes for every birthday and Christmas since I had been ill.

I had been collecting a new wardrobe that I wanted to wear, once I had mastered being able to walk again. I liked to experiment with new styles, because Becky taught me how to express myself through my outfits. Shoes always made me feel like I belong. When I was a teenager at school, the type of trainers you wore determined if you fitted in. Since I first became ill as an inpatient dressed in a gown, I had felt like a bed number, rather than a real person.

I joined the march via Skype and I could see the devastating scenes of the sufferers who had managed to get there. Some were lying on the ground, as the exhaustion stopped them in their tracks. To see people willing to go to this extent made me feel incredibly emotional at the injustice of their suffering.

Hundreds of people sent shoes for the demonstration. Every style of shoe was there; children's ballet shoes represented those missing from their childhood and old shoes showed the lives of those who have passed. There were even a pair of baby booties, to symbolise the children that the M.E. Monster are preventing a sufferer from having. The empty shoes were so poignant because they showed just how many stories of suffering were detached from the real world. This was the only way that our voices could be heard. All those shoes were stuck in a time warp because the world had kept moving, without them.

This level of suffering had to stop. I thought of those words Gran whispered to me, as I was a prisoner in my hospital bed.

"We're going to write that story, Jessica. One day, we'll make your dreams come true."

I had spent years collecting my thoughts on my Dictaphone for the book that I was going to write. I wrote most days, piecing together my life. Samuel came into the room whilst I was contemplating my thoughts about the demonstration I had just witnessed.

He handed me a blue leather book with my initials printed on it in silver. My eyes widened, as I felt the pages with my hands and smelt the familial aroma of a freshly printed book. He'd written a quote inside: *Look at the blank pages before you with courage. Now fill them with beauty.*

"If you're planning to be a published author, then you need a writing book. I know you can't write much at the moment by hand, but it's symbolic. You're a writer!" He smiled at me.

I wrote my name on the first page. This in itself was mind-blowing because in 2007, the first thing that I attempted to do once my arms were straightened from their contraction, was to learn to write again. At first, it was a squiggle but after a lot of practice, I finally wrote *'My name is Jessica and I am going to be an author.'* I couldn't have predicted everything that would happen to get me to this place, but I had always known that I would, somehow, write a book. It was time for my story to be told.

CHAPTER FORTY-FIVE

Chuckles The Chauffeur

Mum was significantly suffering with her health and Becky and Ben had to support her up the stairs after her treatment, where she laid in silence for the rest of the day. All I could hear was her dragging her body to the bathroom, where she would be sick. I felt useless because there was nothing I could do to help.

I tried to send her messages and even FaceTime her upstairs, and she was unrecognisable. I wanted to climb onto the bed and comfort her, as she had spent her life doing for me, but I didn't know any way I could get to her.

My life had been filled with boundaries, and I was used to the Monster forcing me to miss out on everything. But not this time—I had to find a way of getting up those stairs to Mum. I told Samuel how I felt and he suggested picking me up and physically taking me upstairs.

It was the first time I had seen upstairs since the time I lived in my parent's room. My memories of the room were mixed. It was the first place that I managed to sit in a chair. I spent years in there looking at the gap between the curtains, to make out the shape of the trees. I felt strangely detached from the suffering that it reminded me of. I was living a different life now. It was still very limited, but I wasn't quite as imprisoned as I was when I lived there.

Mum was curled on the bed, grey and pale, mirroring me when my health crashed in that room. I just wanted to make her better. I suddenly understood how horrendous it was for my family to watch me be so unwell knowing there was nothing they could do to help. *How had they managed to last over a decade of feeling this helpless?*

I suffered for days for going upstairs but I didn't regret it. At least I got to be with Mum. An agony filled my body from simply being picked up. My seizures increased to a couple of times a week. I hadn't been admitted into hospital with one for a while but they were still immensely disabling. If I overexerted myself, I would have a fit and if I ran on adrenaline for too long, I'd have a convulsion. Anything I did had vast consequences.

Samuel's brother was getting married, and we were invited. Before Tom's wedding and Mum's illness, I would've been resigned to the fact that I'd probably have to miss out on the celebrations, but I felt differently. Sometimes it was worth having the payback if it meant I had wonderful memories and this was one of those moments.

Samuel and I booked into a hotel close to the wedding venue with Dad and my carer. The car was packed with military precision and I was in my wheelchair. Dad was wearing his old ambulance cap from when he had first joined the service.

"Your chauffeur awaits, Jessica," he declared.

I laughed before he wheeled me to the car, telling anyone who would listen that he had decided to retrain as my personal chauffeur. To manage the journey, we stopped regularly, and I had to position my wheelchair horizontally, with no stimulation from music or people talking.

When we arrived, Samuel and Dad lifted me on to the hotel bed, and I laid still for hours. The wedding was in the morning, so I needed to be conscious hours before I would normally be at home. It didn't matter what time I went to sleep, the Monster made sure the mornings were torturous. I had to patiently wait for my energy to reach my body and my medications to work.

Dad came to my room at 8am, and I blearily turned to try and focus on his voice. It echoed around my head, as I tried to make out a coherent sentence.

Dad stroked my hair. "Now, I know Becky christened me with the name Chuckles after the Toy Story 3 clown, and yesterday I turned into Chuckles the Chauffeur. Today, I've got in touch with my feminine side, so you may now know me as Coleen the Hairdresser!" He waved the electric hair curlers in front of me. "Mind you, it's for one day only. Tomorrow I'll revert back to Colin, also known as Chuckles the miserable old git. You can choose which you call me."

Despite doing everything I could to make sure that I paced my energy levels, after being out for half an hour at the ceremony, I needed to lie down. When I entered the reception—hours later—Samuel was talking to his cousin. As soon as he saw me hovering at the door, he brought her over to meet me.

"So lovely to meet you! I can't believe how much this one has changed since being with you. You've been the making of him," she gushed. "Honestly, he used to barricade himself in his room whenever we visited."

I lasted as long as I could at the reception, but I winced in pain as the noise increased. Dad watched as my face drained of colour and excused us. By the time I got to the car, I started to shake uncontrollably as the adrenaline left me to crash.

Once we returned to the hotel, Dad stayed by my side until I drifted off to sleep. A searing agony filled me from electric pain in my legs to a dull ache of exhaustion in every muscle. For the weeks to come, the crash was so extensive, that I struggled to recognise my loved one's voices. That was the torturous reality of the M.E. Monster, when you try to live outside the boundaries it gives you.

Through the suffering, I held on to the special picture that was taken of Samuel and I standing next to each other for a fleeting moment. The Monster didn't always win.

CHAPTER FORTY-SIX

The Art Of De-Ageing

I remembered the day I was diagnosed with severe osteoporosis like it was yesterday. It had been a week before I was due to leave hospital to go home for the first time in four years. I was sent in an ambulance to another hospital for a specialist test on my bones. I wasn't concerned about the scan; I didn't even know what they were looking for.

It had been a gut-wrenching shock when the doctor entered my room and delivered the devastating blow that my bones were riddled with severe osteoporosis. He told me that he was going to start me on treatment straightaway, because my bones were so weak that it was unlikely that I would ever be able to stand up again. I was just nineteen years old and he said that my bones had the density of a one hundred-year old! My world immediately crumbled into pieces. The words he had said on that day still rang in my ears six years later.

Despite being told that there was no way my bones could be fixed, I managed to return to the same hospital years later, and showed the medical team what they said would never happen; I stood up on my own two feet.

Every two years since that first bone density scan there

had been slight gains in my bone density since starting the medication, but it didn't change the prognosis. The truth was any improvement would be something. I couldn't bear the thought of my bones crumbling in my bed, but that was the reality of severe osteoporosis.

It seemed unbelievable that another two years had passed, and I was already on my way to have a repeat Dexa scan done. This time, I was lying down in a recliner wheelchair in the back of my specially adapted car, which we'd lovingly nicknamed 'Brenda Bus.'

I was apprehensive about the scan results, but the actual test was painless. It was the first time that I had made my way to hospital in something other than an ambulance and it was a sign of the progress that I had made over the past two years. It still took a lot of planning; Samuel was in the passenger seat next to my wheelchair with my carer on the other side, to make sure that I didn't lose consciousness or have a seizure.

When I was bed bound, I had to travel forty-five minutes to a hospital that had enough room to facilitate me being on a stretcher. I never understood why all hospitals weren't accessible enough to accommodate patients who couldn't get on to the machine without a hoist. A hospital was meant to look after ill people like me, after all. The fact that I was now able to transfer into a wheelchair for the scan was progress in itself and meant that I could go to the local hospital down the road.

The overstimulating hustle and bustle of people moving in all directions startled me when we arrived. Until then, I had spent most of the time in hospital lying flat and staring at the ceiling, as I hurtled through different corridors in various emergencies.

A bone density scan had the potential to diagnose osteoporosis early. Yet it wasn't protocol for chronically ill people, who were mostly bedridden, to get a scan on the NHS. My bones had weakened extensively due to not being able to weight bear throughout puberty, and if it had been picked up earlier, I may not have be in the position I found myself in.

The only good that came from the ordeal was that other sufferers heard about what happened to me and managed to get a test themselves. I didn't want anyone else to have to be told their bones were beyond repair.

Samuel and Dad lifted me gently out of the wheelchair, so I was standing up. It was an opportune moment to practise moving a few steps without fainting. Although my physio terrorist had been working to increase my standing tolerance, she declared it wasn't safe to do any more exercises until she had seen the results. Everything was riding on this scan, which made me nervous.

The nurse weighed and measured me. My height had significantly increased since I was bedridden. I laid on the scanner, my legs separated by a foam shape. It was over quickly, and it felt strange to think that those two minutes could make or break my dream of walking down the aisle. As I transferred to my wheelchair to go back to the car, I took a deep breath—the wait for the results had begun.

The appointment came for the scan to be reviewed with the osteoporosis team. 'Scaniversaries' brought with them an element of trepidation. It didn't matter what they were scans for.

When we got to the hospital the room was filled with patients suffering from different levels of bone weakness. I signed in and watched the biggest pile of notes move from reception to the nurse practitioner's desk.

"Well, we shall definitely know when it's your turn to be seen!" Samuel whispered into my ear.

I sat in my recliner wheelchair, thinking about what the results would mean for my future. Was it going to be the full stop ending? Or the comma that continued my hope of getting through this?

We waited anxiously for ages for my name to be called. I had always possessed a love for life, and when I was told the news of the severity of the osteoporosis, it stopped me in my tracks. For a while I stumbled, without knowing what to do.

I spent the years that I was in hospital believing that with all the physio terrorist sessions I had endured would help me to get all the range of movement back. The M.E. Monster tried to take everything from me, but it didn't take my hope or belief that this wasn't the way my story ended. . . but the diagnosis of severe osteoporosis was different. It silently crept up on me and shattered my hopes. Even though M.E. was often considered to be an invisible disease, I could still feel the crashes and the agony. Osteoporosis was slowly rotting my bones away, and I didn't feel anything.

"Jessica?" I jumped out of my thoughts, as my name was called.

The nurse ushered Samuel, Dad and I into a small office that could barely fit my wheelchair in. She sat down and looked at my notes. The silence was deafening. After a few minutes, she looked up.

"The good news is your bone scan showed minimal osteoporosis. I think you have mild osteopenia, but whatever you've been doing is working on improving your bones."

I gasped, as I tried to soak in what she said. Samuel squeezed my hand and Dad's mouth fell open.

"So she doesn't have severe osteoporosis? I mean, we were under the impression from the doctors that we spoke to, that it couldn't improve," Dad asked.

Tears of joy filled both mine and Dad's eyes. *How had this happened?*

We fired questions at the nurse, and she smiled at our perplexed faces.

"So, my bones are no longer one hundred years old?" I ask.

"No, they're probably around the same age that you are now." She looked at her notes. "About twenty-five years old, well they might be a bit older than that, but it's nothing you should be terribly concerned with."

"Do I have to stay on the strontium medication?"

"I didn't realise you were on that. Let me ask the consultant." She walked out of the crowded room, and Samuel gave me a big hug.

"I know what this means to you, Jessica. I'm so proud you never gave up."

Dad's hands were frozen to his head, as if he was contemplating the now endless possibilities. We'd spent the past six years resigned to the fact that my bones weren't going to get better. The freedom I felt knowing that the osteoporosis handcuffs were being lifted was overwhelming.

The nurse returned. "Right, so I've been told that you do need to stay on the medication to protect your bones."

"So, why am I still breaking bones?" I asked.

"Your bones are still weaker than they should be. Once you've hurt them, then you have to be a bit more careful. We would expect this from anyone who breaks a bone."

Once we had all our questions answered we prepared to leave. At the door, a sudden burning thought filled me, and I stopped in my tracks. I needed to ask a question that had troubled me desperately since my diagnosis. I remembered that after the doctor had told me the reality of my severe osteoporosis, I had asked him if I would ever be able to have children of my own.

The answer had been a categorical 'no' because my hips were likely to break with the strain. Now, six years later, having done the impossible, did it mean that this had also changed?

"Would I ever be able to have children?" I asked. A silence filled the room.

"I don't see why not. Your bones won't stop you, but your chronic condition might."

Samuel wheeled me outside, where we stopped and tried to take in how much my life had changed after a ten-minute appointment.

I punched my hand in the air and shouted, "Yes! Get in there! I've done it!"

I grabbed my phone to call Mum. She was in London on a day out with Becky, and the two of them cheered, as I screamed down the phone and told them the good news.

Adrenaline filled my body, as I came to terms with the revelation. It took over and I felt like I was riding on cloud nine. The M.E. Monster tried to ruin my day, as an exhaustion filled my brain that meant I needed to lie down. Samuel and

Dad quickly pushed me into the Brenda Bus, as I became paralysed with sheer exhaustion.

"That was too much excitement, honey," Dad soothed, as he attached the seatbelt.

For the next few hours, I laid in the dark in complete silence. I tried to move from side to side to try and get the pain that pulsed into me under control. Even if I managed to get through one of my obstacles, I still had the Monster to contend with. It had already proved to be the longest and most challenging battle that I had ever faced. Dad entered my room holding a drink of whisky in his hand. It wasn't often that you could celebrate such a success in the chronic illness world.

I took hold of the glass and smelt the strong familiar smell of whisky. It reminded me of my childhood, when we had gone on holidays, and had visited the many distilleries that were scattered across Scotland. I took a celebratory gulp of whisky.

"So how does it feel to be younger than you were yesterday?"

"It's very strange. I mean I'm celebrating my bones de-aging!" I said.

"De-aging by seventy-five years to be exact."

"I guess that means today is my minus-seventy-fifth-birthday!"

"To your minus-seventy-fifth-birthday!" Dad and Samuel cheered, and we all took a drink.

I finished the whisky and felt the warm burn in my throat. I was still no fan of the stuff, but I vowed that I would celebrate this day for the rest of my life. The day my body managed the extraordinary. The day that hope came alive again.

CHAPTER FORTY-SEVEN

The Two Faces Of M.E.

Whilst I celebrated the fact that the boundaries of severe osteoporosis had melted away, the M.E. Monster continued to remind me that it was still in control. Although parts of my chronic illness had most definitely improved, it was still frustrating that I could barely leave the confinement of my one room.

I tried to use my social media platform to show an honest account of my life with M.E. but even though I had been running my Facebook page for years, I still struggled to express both faces of the Monster. I showed people when I was managing to do new things, but I wasn't showing how my health could fluctuate so severely within a day.

I hoped that the documentary which I had participated in would help to show that side of the illness. I often spoke to the director to get an update on how the editing was going. It seemed to be taking ages to finish but I knew that the film was going to be part of a global movement to raise awareness of M.E. and that took a long time to plan.

Meanwhile, I was writing my book amid planning a wedding. As I looked through all my entries to my old diary,

Bug, of those horrendous early years in hospital, I was flooded with the memories of everything that had happened. Although I couldn't speak at the time, I knew the title of the book that I planned to write with Gran. She had been my biggest supporter and even though she died a decade ago, it still felt strange to be writing without her.

When I was in hospital my identity had become the dark glasses that I wore, and the M.E. Monster that I lived with. I was a *girl behind dark glasses* and even though my occupational therapist in The Promised Land had called it a 'negative portrayal' all those years ago, I always knew that it was the title I wanted for my book.

The wedding was fast approaching, and I was shocked when I realised that I only had six months to reach my goal of being able to walk down the aisle. My time was split between resting and increasing my core stability, so I would be able to hold myself up. Even though the osteoporosis was not a problem, my body was still much frailer than the average person of my age.

I had been seeing my physio terrorist for three years and I felt safe with her. She worked with my body and she had grown to understand the unpredictability of the Monster. I knew how blessed I was to have a physio terrorist who didn't enforce graded exercise therapy and understood my tolerance levels more than I did. She could even gauge when my blood pressure was beginning to drop. She knew when I needed to stop, even if I didn't say.

It had taken a long time for me to trust a physio terrorist after I spent years being almost bullied into doing exercises and movements that made me feel ill. On the paediatric ward, I was treated like a child with no choice as to how they treated me. The Promised Land wasn't any better and the physio terrorist there would only turn up once in a blue moon leaving my arms to contract. I needed an operation to release them, which was absolute agony.

The physio terrorists at Narnia were lovely and had helped me immensely, but I always suffered long relapses when I returned home due to a lack of available services in the community.

But when my physio terrorist had come into my life, she changed my experience with physiotherapy in the community. She worked my occupational health therapist as a team and had to take on the role of care manager since my last one had left years ago and not been replaced.

She was working hard at creating small exercises that would gently strengthen my body such as Pilates and assisted movements. Our aim was for me to be able to take a few steps at the wedding without collapsing or having an asthma attack. Despite her visiting me fortnightly, we still had a long way to go in six months to achieve that.

One day, she looked troubled when she arrived in my room for one of our appointments. She tried to mask it by reminiscing about the rollercoaster ride we'd been on together, since she had become my physio terrorist.

Something's up she never gets sentimental.

"You know, when I first saw you Jessica, I had no idea if I would ever be able to help you. You collapsed after your head was lifted off the pillow. Now, look at you! It's the proudest I've been." She looked down at the floor with a grimace on her face. "I'm not going to be able to come out to you for much longer.

The bosses have said I've been coming here for too long. The physiotherapy team are only meant to be a short-term service in the community and we're meant to just help people for a few months to get back on their feet, not years."

My mouth fell open, as I tried to digest what she just said. "But how will I even attempt to walk down the aisle with no support? How can you end it now? What about the wedding and the goals we've made?"

I had trusted this physio terrorist implicitly, and I had no doubt that with her, we would be able to make it to the wedding. The hope that had carried me forwards came crashing down. I had tasted a glimpse of what my life could be like, thanks to the determination of this physio terrorist. She helped me sit in a chair for the first time, stabilised my blood pressure and supported me through standing. Now, she was going to be gone. I was alone once more, with so far to go.

I didn't want to spend the rest of my life mostly in bed, looking at the same four walls. My life had all come down to money. In hospital, I was a bed number more than a human and now I was a financial investment rather than a young girl who wanted to live out her potential.

"I just wish I could be treated more like a human with hope, rather than someone with a bloody pound sign on it! I'm worth more than that. I want to be out there, in the world outside my window. You were everything to the progress I've made since you became my physio."

"It's the bosses above me. I must be seen to be reaching targets, that's all they care about. If I don't do that, then I get into trouble and could lose my job."

"I will appeal to your boss," I said desperately. "Give me an email address and I'll do it. They can't just do this! I'll have no support."

My frustration made my heart pummel in my chest, as I tried to take a deep breath. I would have to rely on Team Taylor and Samuel to do everything: from being my carer and nurse to my physiotherapist. There always seemed to be a battle to fight and an injustice to face. I was so tired of it.

The physio terrorist continued with the session. As she moved my limbs to help me stand up I felt numb as I contemplated the fact that this was potentially my last time seeing her. As I tried to stand up, my blood pressure crashed and I overbalanced. She caught me quickly and guided me to the bed as the room around me began to spin. My body was so physically and mentally exhausted. I collapsed before I managed to sit down.

I used up the energy that would've kept me physically standing by getting emotional. I couldn't do both. This was the part of my health that people didn't see. I really did loathe the M.E. Monster for constantly torturing me.

Even though my physio had been told to discharge me, she didn't. She couldn't leave me collapsing, whilst my blood pressure was too low due to physiology. She was concerned that anytime I sat up, it would drop again and take hours to recover. Although I was still going to get sessions, she made it clear that it wouldn't be forever.

It was a juggling act because if I showed too much progress, I would be left, and if I didn't have enough progress, then I had be classed as being too ill to receive help. The local M.E. centre said that I was too ill for support, but my physio was saying I was too well to receive help.

Once she left, I cried with frustration. My life was so uncertain and I felt scared at the complications that I could face from any changes to my routine. Crashes had always led my body to malfunction, but I couldn't cope mentally with the fact that my hopes could be dashed again. I tried to rest so I could recover, but my mind was racing with so many different eventualities that I couldn't emotionally calm down. It was going to be my wedding next year and I didn't want to be left on my own.

My carer made me jump as she entered my room, holding the phone. "It's for you!"

Who was ringing me?

I didn't often receive phone calls, and normally it was only when there was bad news. She was grinning as she handed me the phone.

"Hello?"

"Hi Jessica, I'm a reporter from the Medway Messenger. I just wanted to congratulate you because you've been nominated for the Pride in Medway Award by your pharmacist."

I was dumbfounded. My pharmacist had never met me in person, but I spoke to her often about my medications. She would always ask about everything I did, but I had no idea it was for this. I listened to the reporter on the other end of the phone while a million thoughts passed through my mind. Amidst my dampened faith in bureaucracy, it made me realise that people did care.

After the phone call, I laid still in my one room. Instead of fighting the exhaustion like I had a tendency to try to do, I had to co-exist with the Monster: my body needed to rest.

I woke up hours later to the sound of music coming from

the other room. Becky was playing on the piano and I longed to join her. I wanted to have a moment to immerse myself in the world of music, where I didn't have to hurt anymore.

I asked my carer to push me into the living room in my wheelchair so I could listen to Becky play. As I watched her fingers move on the white and black keys, I imagined that it was me.

Becky turned around and smiled at me. "It's about time that you actually sat at the piano."

She got up and came to my wheelchair to help me stumble to the stool with my carer. I closed my eyes and the music flowed through me. My fingers started to dance, as they remembered how to play the tune I had last played before the Monster had pounced. All my worries eroded away, as I became lost in the moment, with the power of music, despite my noise sensitivity, it made everything seem okay.

When I returned to my bed ten minutes later, I was smiling. I sat up in bed dancing to mine and Samuel's song. I felt carefree for a moment. I only moved my hands, but the music magically spoke to me in a way words couldn't.

An hour later, the jubilation drained from me as the M.E. Monster crashed down. The exhaustion suffocated me. Samuel tried to comfort me, but the words I tried to say back were incomprehensible. I tried to curl up in a ball, but I was in searing agony. My speech slurred; my groans were my only way of conversing that I was in pain. Samuel sat in the bed next to me and held me to him. In a short space of time, I was a completely different person, battling to be able to stay conscious.

They were the two faces of the M.E. Monster who controlled

my entire life. The post-exertional malaise I suffered from playing the piano was extensive. All I could do was focus on surviving through every hour of the day, with Samuel nursing me through the hurricane crash I faced for trying to live.

A year had passed since Mum received her cancer diagnosis. A whole year of treatment and constant suffering. Unfortunately, her last scan had shown that her cancer had metastasized to other parts of her body. Thankfully, she was having a break from her radiotherapy sessions over the Christmas holidays, which meant she was in good spirits.

She found activities exhausting and we felt like we understood each other in a way no one else could. The tiredness Mum felt was a similar fatigue that blighted me. The only difference was my exhaustion stayed with me—I hadn't been able to get away from it for ten years.

We wanted to make my last Christmas as a Taylor count, so Mum got lots of tacky festive décor for us to wear with our Christmas jumpers for a family photo. For the first time in years, we had a Christmas without medical emergencies or trips to hospital.

My family didn't know what to do with themselves, as there was no stress! The biggest drama was Dad burning the roast potatoes; the air went blue with expletives. Becky and Ben helped him forget all about it by getting him to taste their homemade gin. It didn't take long before we'd all given it a try.

Samuel came into our room in the evening and shut the door. He lit some candles all around the darkened room and put on our favourite Christmas songs for us to sing along to. We may have sounded out of tune as we belted out the songs to each other, but we didn't care. When *Walking in the Air* came on, Samuel took to miming rather than singing and I conducted him whilst in hysterics.

"I can't wait to marry you next year, Jessica," he said, as he cuddled into me.

"Me neither!" I whispered in his ear.

On New Year's Eve, Samuel and I counted down the hours to midnight and the beginning of 2017—the year that was going to completely change both of our lives. Although the fireworks were already giving me a headache, I couldn't help but feel excited for the year to come. The documentary film that I was featured in would be released in a few weeks, I was going to marry my best friend, and we would be crowdfunding to bring my book *A Girl Behind Dark Glasses* to life.

My hope to be able to walk down the aisle was very much alive. I had been following a gentle plan that my physio terrorist had given me to help my autonomic system cope when I stood up. She couldn't see me as often as she used to, as she was still fighting her bosses, but she trained my carers to be able to do the exercises safely when she wasn't there.

Everything was going to plan, and I knew I had to be extra careful to make sure that I looked after my body enough because I couldn't afford a setback. No matter what my health was like, I found that I always dipped into a setback after the festive period.

2017

CHAPTER FORTY-EIGHT

Weebles Wobble But They Don't Fall Over

On the first Sunday of the New Year, Samuel cuddled up to me on my bed to watch the third series of *Sherlock* together. I loved watching the clever storytelling and how the actors had modernised the characters to perfection.

I was caught up in the moment of watching an intricate plotline coming alive when I absentmindedly rolled over to grab a drink from the side. It still felt incredible to be able to do that without having to even think about it anymore. I wasn't watching where I was going because my eyes were glued to the television screen. I didn't want to miss anything!

In a split second of wrong judgement, I overcooked the turn and to my horror began to overbalance. I was crashing straight out of the bed. It happened with a mixture of speed and slow motion. I could feel myself falling further than I had done before. It was as if I was on the edge of a rollercoaster that was about to drop. The floor now seemed incredibly close and I knew there was nothing I could do to prevent the inevitable from occurring.

An ear-piercing scream filled the house and it took me a while to realise the noise was coming from me. I hurtled over the edge of the bed and fell on to the cold, hard, floor. My head hit first, followed by a horrendous noise as the rest of my body crashed down.

Samuel darted out of the bed to reach me, but it was too late. My body was in severe pain. Mum and Dad came running to see what the commotion was and gasped at my body crumpled on the ground.

The immediate damage consisted of a twisted neck, sore hip, and bruised knee. The problem was, I had no means of getting back into bed. My parents assessed how I could be moved without causing further problems. The floor was freezing and despite being in pain, my body continued to shiver in shock.

It took four people to be able to lift me up from the floor. A carry sheet was placed underneath my body enabling them to safely lift me. I continued to shake uncontrollably and my pain levels tripled. Once I was transferred safely into my bed, the cot sides trapped me to prevent another fall.

Shit! Had I just completely thrown away my plans for the wedding? Never mind walking, would I even be able to get there? What the hell was I going to do?

Samuel could see the fear in my eyes, and he grabbed hold of my hand. "Jessica, don't panic. You've put so much into your plan into our wedding and you'll get there. Give yourself some time."

"I. . . I. . . can't give myself time. I've been reaching for this goal for the past year and now everything is lost."

"It's not lost, I promise. If it had happened this time last year, then I would agree with your fears. But think about it, you've just had a scan that has shown you're no longer suffering with severe osteoporosis. You've never fallen before, have you?" Samuel said.

I gave a weakened smile, as I realised that I couldn't move my neck without suffering from shooting pain.

"Imagine if this had happened when you had severe osteoporosis. You would have probably broken your spine and pelvis. So, this is okay. You need to take some pain relief and I'll get the ice packs to stop the swelling."

He always managed to calm me down when I was overwhelmed. It was a blip, just like Samuel said. I just wondered if we would both be saying the same thing in the next couple of days when the bruising came out.

I woke up in the morning to find that I was covered in them from head to toe. I had to keep myself focused on anything other than the pain I was in. The final parts to the wedding were being planned and the designer inside of me came out to play. We were going to transform the little village hall into something miraculous. There was a starry backdrop that was able to twinkle effervescently and Samuel's mum was making lines of bunting. Everything was planned meticulously with the help of our family and friends.

My physio terrorist came to assess the damage I had done to myself from the fall. As she looked at every part of my body, a furrow appeared in between her eyebrows.

"It's not great but it could've been a lot worse."

I let out a sigh of relief. She asked my carer to give me some pain relief, so she could begin to mobilise my joints. It was a matter of rest and recuperation, whilst she manipulated my body to fix it.

Over the next couple of weeks she came to see me more

often, because it was important to keep my body moving through the pain I was in, so that I could eventually get up again. Even though I tried to keep going through the agony, my body was beginning to struggle.

"Jessica, I think we need to change our tactics. I don't think we should push your body anymore. Your M.E. does not deal well with being forced to do something. I think that sounds a bit like graded exercise, and you said that made you worse."

It was a phenomenal difference to have a healthcare professional who made a point of listening to what I told her. I felt sad because I knew that what she said was true; it was about working with my body through this setback.

Ever since I first became unwell, I pinned all my hopes on achieving a single goal. At times, it worked in my favour but when I didn't achieve what I set out to do, it made me struggle mentally with the everyday traumas that the M.E. Monster put me through.

It was a dangerous way of dealing with this horrendous disease, but it had been part of my coping mechanism. It had always given me something to think about whilst I was trapped in my own surroundings. The M.E. Monster didn't work with plans. It didn't do what I told it to. I knew that my idea of walking down the aisle wasn't worth the constant paralysis I was suffering. It was hard to come to terms with, but I knew that as long as I got to marry Samuel that was all that mattered. It would just be an added bonus if I did manage to walk.

CHAPTER FORTY-NINE

Time For Unrest

Whilst I recovered from my fall, I was given the opportunity to watch a copy of the film documentary I featured in, *Unrest*, before its premiere at the Sundance Festival. It had followed my journey with the M.E. Monster for the past four years. The film was trying to speak universally—you didn't need to know about the reality of the M.E. Monster to understand the story it was trying to tell. The important thing was the campaign surrounding the film had the potential of getting people talking about M.E. and I was so ready for that conversation to start.

Mum and Dad watched the film with me in total silence. It was overwhelming to see how the film, which told the stories of five M.E. sufferers, intricately weaved them together so beautifully. My life had changed so much in the past four years since the filming took place that I felt detached from the 'me' in the film.

When I saw myself, I looked like a stranger. I had started the process lying flat in my hospital bed, unable to sit up and had finished with me standing for a few minutes. I now had new challenges and isolations to face that were a far cry away from what my situation was in the film.

The film showed how much we desperately needed visibility and research into the M.E. Monster. It needed to be more than just sufferers fighting for a change. At that moment, the treatment was dependant on the lottery of where you lived in the world. It seemed impossible that we were in the twenty-first century, and still people were being forcibly removed from their homes to institutions. Becoming unwell was the only reason for their punishment.

It made me realise how lucky I had been to receive support from different teams both at Narnia and in the community. It had most certainly been a rocky road to find the right help, but it reinstated my fear of losing it in the future.

Mum's scan at the beginning of the year revealed that the cancer had started to spread even further. She was started on a harsher treatment, but she still managed to carry on, despite her suffering. She would sit for hours talking to me about what I was planning to do with my hair and makeup for the wedding. It kept her fighting. She wanted to be well enough to enjoy the day.

It was hard to see her struggle, because physically she was managing but mentally, she wasn't. On top of that, she had been panicking about me ever since my fall. She spent her life protecting me, at first as a mother to a defenceless baby, all the way up to a vulnerable adult. It had given her a purpose, but now Samuel was able to look after me, it made her feel like her health problems were taking me away from her.

In a way, I understood her thinking. Becky now spent her time looking after Mum. As the dynamic had shifted and as wonderful as it was to have Samuel taking over my care, it felt like Becky had been taken away from me.

The wedding felt like it was really happening when my dress arrived. I hadn't been able to go to a shop to try on any dresses, so Becky and Mum helped me shop online. We sat together with a cup of tea and some chocolate to make it feel special as we scoured the internet to find the 'one.' Being disabled made it more of a challenge because the dress had to fit a certain criteria. I had to be able to sit for long periods in my wheelchair without running over it, and it had to be easy to walk in.

Mum always had an eye for finding dresses that fitted my style. She always brought home incredible clothes for me that she found whilst volunteering at the charity shop. I could never understand how she managed to do it.

She came across a website that had all sorts of wedding dresses for very reasonable prices. As we were going to have to order one and then try it on, we didn't want to waste any money with expensive ones. I watched over her shoulder, as she scrolled through the pages. Then I saw it. . . that was the one! It was ivory with a sweetheart neckline and sparkled with sequins across the bodice.

Becky and Mum helped me to squeeze it on whilst lying down. They helped me to my feet, and were both overcome with emotion as I stood up. When I looked in the mirror, I immediately felt like it was perfect; it looked beautiful.

At that moment, I was suddenly hit by an acceptance that I hadn't felt before. I looked down at my body, as it shook with the sheer effort of holding itself up and smiled. In the past few months, I had constantly been trying to achieve a 'normal' life of having my dream wedding and walking down the aisle. But it wasn't about that, it was about marrying the man I loved. Even if I didn't manage to walk, that was okay.

My body had survived through the unimaginable. I mean it was a miracle that I could even stand up!

The build-up to all my past achievements had been immense. They were huge moments in my life, but the actual successes had passed in seconds. I had never really been able to accept before that my body might not achieve what I had set out to do.

The first time I sat in a chair had been years in the making. My body hadn't managed it straight away, but I saw that as part of the journey. I always believed that I would succeed in doing it. I hadn't given myself the chance to accept that my future would stay in one room, because I mentally couldn't cope with that. Every goal had been stressful. I had pushed my body to its limits and crashed horrendously afterwards, often ending up relapsing and being rushed into hospital.

But this was different, I wanted to enjoy the wedding; it was about me and Samuel and our commitment to each other. I didn't have to prove anything to anyone anymore, including myself. I wanted to learn to live *with* the M.E. Monster, not fight *against* him.

No matter what happened, it was going to be a day of celebration. I laid down to rest and felt the pain ease as my body began to relax into the mattress. Taking the pressure off myself was going to make the lead up a complete joy. It was going to be my last few months of being a Taylor and it was the start of a new adventure.

With the wedding fast approaching everything we planned seemed to be falling into place. We only had a small budget to spend and it really felt like it was being arranged by the whole community—the church had waivered the fee, my grandad would play the organ, and Elizabeth planned to sing at the reception, whilst her mum did all the food. To keep it personal, we asked both of our brothers to be ushers, along with my old friend Nick and Becky's boyfriend Ben. Stewie was going to be the best man, and I had Becky as chief bridesmaid with my two old friends, Kara and Harriet.

The colour theme was going to be a range of different blues. The bridesmaid dresses were a striking blue, the ushers were in navy suits with grey waistcoats, whilst Samuel and Stewie were going to be in the opposite. We managed to get hold of blue ribbon to decorate Brenda Bus, and we had a driver that would take Mum and the bridesmaids in his stunning classic car for free.

Becky had been organising my Hen Do for ages, so the last thing that I needed to do was see whether I would be well enough to attempt any steps to walk down the aisle. My physio terrorist had been trying to strengthen my injured body from the fall. She even visited the church in Upnor where we planned to get married, to plot out the exact number of steps to the altar. Even though she managed to shorten the length of the aisle with the vicar, I still needed to walk twelve steps and there was a small part of me that hoped I could do it.

CHAPTER FIFTY

The Hen Do

Becky's plan for the Hen Do was to make it accessible and fun, whilst ensuring it didn't affect my health too much. She decided to split it into two parts to enable me to have all my friends there without it being too overwhelming. I just couldn't manage lots of people in one room at the same time. It was exhausting to see different faces, start new conversations and then try and do activities. Becky was adamant that the Hen Do would be something that suited my needs. She spent days locked up in her room organising everything.

"All you need to know is your Hen Do will be incredible. Inclusive, because we're doing it at home, and you will be able to lay flat. Fun, because I mean, I'm organising it and it will include your favourite thing like *Harry Potter.* It will be a HP extravaganza. Then, I thought we would have to cater for the churchy peeps, who probably won't enjoy the whole HP world, so part two of your hen do will be a *Winnie the Pooh* afternoon tea. The rest of my plans are shrouded in secrecy. So you'll have to wait!"

On the day of the Hen Do Part One, my carer helped me change into a costume that Becky had prepared for me days before. I groaned as I saw the horrendous clothes that she had chosen. They were at least double the size of me and she had put a sumo wrestle fat suit in with the outfit. The only *Harry Potter* character that I could think of was Harry's horrible Aunt Marge, the one who Harry blows up!

"Oh yes!" Becky entered the room to find me in the fat suit. "Now you need to have buttons that can fall off as you inflate."

Only then did I notice Becky's attire. She had fully gone for the fancy-dress theme. She had dressed up as Hedwig, Harry's snowy owl. Every time she moved, she spread her fabric wings and made a hoot. Honestly!

Whilst my friends started to arrive, I laid in the pitch black to rest as much as I could before the party started. Everyone was seated in the living room, awaiting my entrance, Becky squeezed my hand tightly.

"Now you see, if I wasn't going as Aunt Marge from Harry Potter, you would have totally won the best costume design!" I said, as she hooted in response.

My head was already beginning to feel heavy from the adrenaline as I listened to the voices of the guests. I had not had this many people in my house since before I was ill. It was exhausting just trying to think of what I was going to say to everyone.

Don't get me wrong, it was exciting, but my energy tended to be zapped out of me so quickly that I had no control over what happened. I took a deep breath, knowing the hours of preparation Becky had put into the hen do.

She caught my face and smiled understandingly. "If it's too much, then you can just go back to your room."

I knew that this was the chance to see how my sensory sensitivities were doing.

I had spent the past few months slowly increasing the number of stimuli I could tolerate, ready for the overload I was going to experience on the wedding day. It had started off with listening to music loudly, then I had watched television to try to improve my concentration when listening to lots of people talking together.

I was hoisted into my specialist reclining chair (my costume made it difficult to squeeze into!) and wheeled out into the dining room. I gulped, as I saw that it had been transformed into the great hall of Hogwarts, with floating candles made out of toilet rolls. It had been planned with such attention to detail and looked incredible. I marvelled at all the decorations, as I was slowly moved into the living room. It was full of my close friends, who all looked up from their conversations as they saw me.

There was a unanimous cry of laughter, as Becky pressed the fat suit that was under my ghastly outfit and I began to inflate.

For the next hour and a half, I laughed more than I had for a long time. The door to the hallway had been covered with a brick poster to mimic platform 9 and ¾ and we had an absolute blast as I lived my childhood dream of entering Hogwarts, albeit from my own house. It was the first time I had spent time with my school friends and cousins in years. I was back to my jokester self, laughing and chatting like old times. We played quizzes and we ate chocolate frogs to our hearts' desires.

In what felt like no time at all, I could feel myself beginning to fade. The adrenaline that had got me through the past hour and a half left me, and the neurological symptoms came flooding back into view.

Becky saw and helped me make a quick exit back to my room. She and my carer hoisted me back into the bed, where I laid silently. My body ached. I was so exhausted that I couldn't rest.

Samuel entered the room and just held my hand, until I began to drift off to sleep. As I turned over, Samuel whispered, "Did you enjoy it?"

With every last bit of energy, I murmured, "Today was a good day."

And the lights went out. I returned to Limbo Land.

The days after the Hen Do Part One had been difficult. It was hard to always pay for every single thing that I did. I was so proud that I had managed to stay for as long as I did, but now was the time to rest. I didn't have long, because in a few weeks, I would be going back to the living room to join in with a different set of friends for Part Two.

The theme was *Winnie the Pooh*, another all-time favourite. I remembered listening to *The House at Pooh Corner* on cassette, with Stephen Fry voicing Winnie the Pooh and Dame Judi Dench voicing Piglet. The actual Hundred Acre Wood was not far from my home, and I had spent many an afternoon playing Pooh Sticks in the stream.

I held on to these happy memories as I suffered with inordinate amounts of pain and exhaustion that made it hard to focus on anything happening within my little world. My only activity was the gentle physiotherapy exercises to improve my autonomic system for the big day.

My physio terrorist had calculated that I needed to be able

to stand for approximately eight minutes altogether. With just one month left to go, I could stand for six minutes before I went lightheaded and had to be guided to my bed.

The second part of the Hen Do wasn't going to be very taxing. Instead of dressing up, Becky insisted that we would only play small games. Part Two was for the more mature ladies, my Mum, Samuel's Mum, plus my family friends from church who weren't particularly interested in *Harry Potter*. It was going to be a lot of fun and I was looking forward to the socialising.

On the morning of Part Two, my carer helped me do my makeup. I went into hibernation mode before the party, with people only entering to give me more medication and food.

I wanted to eat before the party because I was still slightly embarrassed that I couldn't yet feed myself a full meal independently. Having rested and prepared, I felt a bit more comfortable and confident as I was hoisted back into the chair. This was going to be okay because it wasn't going to be nearly as strenuous as Part One.

I had a whale of a time with everyone, as we played traditional party games. Becky put us into teams and the goal was to make a wedding dress out of toilet paper. A simple but hilarious task.

I should have noticed then as the Monster seeped into every cell. I should've stopped there, but I wanted to have some fun with my friends. I rebelled for half an hour longer before my carer wheeled me back into my room.

Then it started.

I couldn't get out of the chair. I didn't have the energy to hold my head up to be hoisted back to the bed. I could feel my energy wasting away and there was nothing I could do. The carer shouted out for help and two people hurried over. I couldn't even tell who they were. My vision was blurry. Everything hurt. To breathe, to think, to hope.

Hours later, I awoke from my crash, but it was not over. I could feel someone holding my hand and softly stroking my face. It took me a while to realise it was Samuel. I tried to talk to him, but nothing came out. I tried again and a few incoherent noises surfaced but he couldn't understand me. It felt as though I was drowning in a current of exhaustion. I had nothing more to give, and I fell into Limbo Land.

I drifted in and out of consciousness and panicked when I couldn't communicate back to Samuel. My body shook uncontrollably, as it whimpered in suffering. I felt the worst that I had felt in the past year, and I was going to be getting married in a month. Everything had changed in the space of a few fragile minutes. One afternoon had made all the difference.

Was I willing to sacrifice this much for one day?

Tears filled my eyes, as I tried to gain back some form of control and turn the lights in my brain back on. They didn't budge for days.

Was it going to be possible to go to my own wedding day? Let alone walk down the aisle?

Samuel spent the next week constantly caring for me as I slept through the days, waking only for more pain relief.

I had to hold on with everything that I had as the hurricane devastated my body. It was scary to see the deterioration happen so quickly, and to not know when I would be able to resurface again.

In the moments that I was able to think, I thought of what

I was going to do. I had to focus on each breath, inhaling and exhaling slowly. As Samuel held my hand, I was reminded of how Gran had always held it like that when I had been suffering. In the moments that I was awake, I moved my fingers and fiddled with my rings. The opal ring that had been Gran's was on my right and I felt the diamonds of my engagement ring on my wedding finger. It gave me strength through my pain.

Over the next few days, I started to pull through the crash. It had given me a new sense of what the consequences of this goal could be for my body. Even though I wanted it so much, I decided that what would be, would be. I was powerless to the Monster, and I needed just to survive.

I spent the time dreaming of the special day. I let my mind linger on the beautiful countryside that I had seen when I had visited the church months before. The sun had been shining that day and the fields that surrounded the church were full of yellow flowers. I had three weeks to recover from the blip. All I could do was give my body the best chance.

The physio terrorist came to visit me and ordered bed rest until the day of the wedding.

"You've done everything you possibly can. We now need to work *with* your body, not against it. It's telling you to rest. Don't panic, it's going to work out."

I nodded my head as she spoke.

Come on body, you can do this, I thought desperately.

"I'm proud of you whatever happens," Samuel said. "It will all be fine."

All I could do was believe him, as he believed in me.

CHAPTER FIFTY-ONE

Love Shine A Light

From the beginning, Samuel and I wanted to involve all our friends in our wedding. Whilst we had physical friends, the online community had also made such a big impact on our lives. Without the internet, we would have never met; it had been instrumental in our relationship, and it was a lifeline for the chronically ill community.

There were many who lived too far or weren't well enough to make the journey to the church. We wanted to find a way to make them involved in our special day.

A couple of months before the wedding, I was particularly struggling with my light sensitivity. Any form of light was incredibly painful, so I laid in the pitch-black darkness. Samuel lit a candle, and we watched as the light banished the darkness.

A candle had been the one thing that had always been present in my life. Gran always lit candles to show she was thinking of someone. Whenever I had a problem, she would always say, "Let me light you a candle, darling."

To see that spark in a darkened world was comforting. Back at the beginning of my diagnosis, a candle had been my only source of light in my room. Throughout my journey, it acted as a beacon of hope for me.

Gran had always said that when you lit one candle, it would light up the world. Throughout my illness, she always asked her friends to light a candle. On my sixteenth birthday, Mum told her that I was particularly unwell, so she lit her living room up with sixteen candles, to make sure I knew that I wasn't alone.

As I thought of those memories, the idea of getting all our friends to light a candle on the day of our wedding came to me. Candles were universal and no matter where everyone was in the world, they could all be a part of our day.

Samuel started a campaign to spread the message amongst the M.E. community and our friends. The response was incredible! There were people contacting us from Australia, Norway, Germany and America, to name a few. It felt completely overwhelming to think that so many people wanted to light candles and become part of our celebration. I guess love really does shine a light.

The day had arrived! I had celebrated 29th April for the whole of my existence. This date would have been my Gran's seventy-seventh birthday. Yet she was now only a vivid memory, which I held close to me. When I closed my eyes, I felt like I could almost touch her. I could feel her immaculate skin on my fingertips and hold her hands. I closed my eyes for a little longer, holding on to Gran in every inch of my mind.

"You're getting there, darling."

I imagined that I could hear her whisper to me, the same words she had said to me nine years ago. I held her memory closely, and I visualised myself leaning on her shoulder, and wrapping my arms around her like old times.

"Look at you!" I pictured her saying to me. "You have such a bright future, darling one. You're just lovely. Always remember that."

"Happy birthday Gran," I whispered to her.

In my mind, she stopped me and smiled effervescently. "We share this day now."

I just wanted to hear her voice on repeat, but I knew she wasn't really there. My heart broke into pieces to think that she wouldn't be here to witness my wedding. All I could do was imagine her with all the other people I had lost along the way.

"Happy wedding day, sweetheart. I love you."

And with that I opened my eyes from my quiet reverie, ready to face the day that would change my life forever and pave the way for my future. Dad came into the room, bringing the blind up.

"You ready little one?"

I looked up at the sky from my bed, which was the brightest blue with the sun glistening brightly. I closed my eyes for one more moment and could see the image of Gran nodding encouragingly at me.

"You bet I am, Dad."

He gave me a hug and I saw to my delight that he had lit a tea light candle in my room. I was ready for this moment.

In no time, people started to arrive, from my school friend who was doing the pre-wedding photography, to my hairdresser and the makeup artist—not to mention all the bridesmaids.

I was marrying the man of my dreams and it felt like the whole of Kent had come together to make this day possible.

My phone continued to buzz, as the day dawned all over the world and people sent me pictures of the candles they had lit. There were so many positive messages of hope coming from America to Australia and everywhere in between.

I tried to soak up the relaxed atmosphere from my bed because I knew that today I was going to be starting a new chapter as a married woman. I knew that life was such an incredible gift, and to have someone to share every moment with meant I was the luckiest girl on the planet, despite the adversity I had faced.

Ever since I had first become unwell at fifteen, I had chosen to fight this illness with everything that I had. It had been a tumultuous journey over the past eleven years, but as I laid in my bed listening to the excited bridal party, I thought of all the achievements I had made in that time.

The moment I had first seen my face without my dark glasses on was so huge! I hadn't recognised myself. After two years of being unable to speak, I had fought for my voice to be able to communicate.

Despite the awful carer, Jackson, who abused me whilst I was in hospital, with taunts that I would never be listened to, I had pushed for people to hear me. The euphoria I felt when I finally managed to scratch the itch on the end of my nose was immeasurable. The elation I felt when I had first sat in a chair for five seconds was out of this world.

To do something as normal as rolling over in bed when I was uncomfortable felt like such a privilege after years of being stuck flat on my back. Doctors had disbelieved me, as they were sure I would never be able to stand up again, but I had gone and done it.

I had gone and done it!

As the magical day unfolded, I momentarily felt the losses that I had gone through, too. My Gran had died, as did my dad's father, Grampy, and again I had to miss his funeral. The devastating truth was he'd never seen his granddaughter talk again. I was too unwell to say goodbye.

M.E. had caused dismay and a level of suffering that was incomprehensible. Even on my wedding day, I was thwarted by an agony and exhaustion that filled every cell in my body.

The hairdresser came into my room and started to plait my long locks softly around the side of my head and into a bun. My tiara was filled with sparkling beads, and when it was placed on my head, it looked perfect, just as I had envisaged it would be.

I wore Mum's delicate pearl teardrop earrings, and the makeup gave me a welcome glow to my usually pale complexion. The florist knocked on the door and showed me the beautiful bouquet of blue and cream flowers, she had put together. I attached three small frames around the stems with pictures of my grandparents who were no longer with us: Gran, Grandma, and Grampy. They would be with me as Dad gave me away.

The bridesmaids changed into their gowns, and Samuel's three-year-old god sister, was our little flower girl. She was a bundle of energy, as she pranced around in her cream dress with blue flowers. Everything looked so perfect and exactly as I had imagined. To conserve my energy, I laid quietly in a room until the very last moment. With just ten minutes to spare, my carer helped me quickly change into my ivory dress.

For the first time, I stood up and saw myself. I looked beautiful. Mum entered my room exactly at that moment and her face lit up. The smile that filled her face masked the intense pain she was in. Today, her cancer was not going to win. Not even the M.E. Monster was going to get an edge in.

This was *our* day, and no matter what happened, nothing was going to take that away from us. We cried as we embraced tightly. Once Dad, Tom, and Becky entered my room we had a moment of holding each other's hands. This had been such a long time in the making.

As I got ready to leave, the emotion got to me. My life had been made up of these four walls. This room had been my only existence and it felt utterly overwhelming to be leaving it when I knew that everything was going to change for the better. I was ready to meet Samuel for the beginning of the rest of our lives.

When Mum and Becky brought the wheelchair into my room, I gasped.

"We thought it needed to be jazzed up for the occasion, so we added some flowers," Mum said.

"Look at the lights Blissy sent me to put on," Becky added as she pointed to the blue and white lights around the wheels.

I thought of my dearest Blissy who I had asked her to be my 'bedbound bridesmaid' because I knew she wouldn't be well enough to physically come. The fact that she was still a big part of my day meant so much. I took one last moment to check my phone to see the mass of messages that had been sent to me, with pictures of the candles that were lit across the world.

I had given myself the best shot. I had worked on small exercises over the past year to plan meticulously for every possible outcome. I was as ready as I would ever be. The adrenaline pumped through my veins, and that was the only thing keeping me going as we reached the church.

The little country church was full to the brim with all my friends and family. This was the moment I had been waiting for. Tom pushed my wheelchair into the porch of the church, where Dad and Becky were ready to help me to my feet.

I peered into the congregation and couldn't help but smile at what I saw. Everyone turned around to watch me with bated breath, while Becky and Dad held me steady. Then the music began to play.

Any sound caused me a great deal of pain, so I had stuffed my ears with earplugs to try and muffle it. Through the discomfort, Dad squeezed my shoulder to check that I was okay, and I nodded gently towards him. This was it.

Dad held me tight and we began to walk forwards towards the aisle. I focused on looking ahead of me, and I pushed my legs to move independently. I could feel my muscles heave on my legs and it took all the energy that I had. The longest walk I had made in eleven years began. To my exhilaration, I started to put one step in front of the other, and slowly walked towards Samuel.

As I moved past each pew, the row would stand up, so I would not to be overwhelmed by everyone. The Monster that had dictated what I was able to do for so many years, was shrouded by all the candles and people's thoughts that were alight.

I started to feel out of breath as we reached the halfway point. I wasn't used to moving so far. With just a couple of steps to go, adrenaline filled my body and it carried me the rest of the way. I was ushered over to the special chair that had been kept in the church for me to recline in.

My family sat in the nearest pew to me, so they could assist me at any moment if needed. Their eyes were trained for the very smallest motion that looked like I was going to collapse. I looked around at the packed little church, then I looked at Samuel and at the vicar who was smiling at me. The relief flooded over me at the realisation that I had done it. I had managed to walk down the aisle!

"You made it then," Samuel whispered into my ear as he took hold of my hand.

After I had collected myself together, we stood up for our vows. I couldn't believe that I had finally managed to end this chapter, and as I uttered the words, "I do," I looked at everyone watching.

Dr Nice had his hand held up to his face. Without Dr Nice, I would never have made it to this day. There were so many obstacles in my way, and he was hands-down the only doctor in my journey who continually believed in me. I caught his eye and he smiled and gave a little nod.

"I pronounce you man and wife," the vicar announced.

Applause filled the church and I looked back at Samuel. My best friend and now my husband. He squeezed my hand, as the full magnitude of what we had done filled us both. He led me back down the aisle. I was floating on cloud nine.

As I reached the porch, I collapsed into my wheelchair. The adrenaline made my body shake uncontrollably with relief. I couldn't ask anything more of my body. It had done more than I could ever have hoped for.

The M.E. Monster tried to rear its ugly head, but it could not be heard over the celebrations.

About the Author

Jessica Taylor-Bearman is the number 1 bestselling author of *A Girl Behind Dark Glasses* which shares her real life experience with living with M.E (Myalgic Encephalomyeletis). *A Girl Behind Dark Glasses* has stayed on the bestsellers list since its release in 2018.

Jessica was born in 1991 in Kent. She lived a very active life until she became seriously unwell with M.E. when she was fifteen-years-old. She has spent a vast amount of time in hospital due to the severity of her illness and was completely bed bound for over a decade.

Whilst in hospital, Jessica spent her time coming up with ideas of how she could help others. She is the founder of Share a Star, a charity that helps seriously unwell youngsters. She writes a blog called *The World of One Room* and has a YouTube video of the same name that has reached tens of thousands of people in multiple countries. Jessica has also featured in an Oscar-nominated film *Unrest*. She is an advocate for raising awareness of M.E. and has spoken at the Houses of Parliament.

She lives with her husband in Essex and welcomed her miracle daughter Felicity in 2019. She now tries to raise awareness of chronically ill and disabled mums, with the hope of making the world that little bit more accessible.

Find out more at www.jaytay.co.uk
Follow her on Twitter @jayletay
Instagram @jayletay
Facebook.com/TheWorldOfOneRoom